Socioeconomic Status and Adolescent Well-being

Ahmed Siddiqui

Unauthorized use of this material is strictly prohibited.
Copyright © 2023, Ahmed Siddiqui. All rights reserved.

CONTENT

CHAPTER 1	INTRODUCTION	1-21
1.1	Origin of the study	11
1.2	Significance of the study	14
1.3	Statement of the problem	17
1.4	Delimitations	18
1.5	Functional and operational definition of the key terms	18
	1.5.1 Socio-economic status	18
	1.5.2 Self-confidence	18
	1.5.3 Mental health	19
	1.5.4 Personal values	19
	1.5.5 Adolescent	20
1.6	Objectives of the study	20

CHAPTER 2	REVIEW OF LITERATURE	22-46
2.1	**STUDIES ON SOCIO-ECONOMIC STATUS**	22
	1. Socio-economic status and health	23
	2. Socio-economic status and achievement	24
	3. Socio-economic status and self-confidence	27
	4. Socio-economic status and mental health	28
	5. Socio-economic status and personal values	30
2.2	**STUDIES ON SELF-CONFIDENCE**	31
	1. Locality, school and gender difference among adolescents self-confidence.	31
	2. Self-confidence and academic achievement.	33
	3. Self-confidence and mental health	34
2.3	**STUDIES ON MENTAL HEALTH**	36
	1. Locality, school and gender difference among adolescents mental health	36
	2. Mental health and academic achievement	38
	3. Emotional maturity and emotional stability	39
	4. Adjustment level	41
2.4	**STUDIES ON PERSONAL VALUES**	42
	1. Effect of personal values	42
	2. Academic achievement and personal values	43
	3. Locality, gender difference and type of school among adolescents personal values	43
2.5	**HYPOTHESIS OF THE STUDY**	45

CHAPTER 3	DESIGN OF THE STUDY	47-67
3.1	Research questions	47

3.2	Method of the study		47
3.3	Population		47
3.4	Sample and sampling technique		53
3.5	Variables of the study		55
3.6	Tools used		55
	3.6.1 Modified kuppuswamy's SES scale		55
	3.6.2 Self-Confidence inventory		57
	3.6.3 Personal value scale		58
	3.6.4 Mental health battery		62
3.7	Administration of test		66
3.8	Statistical techniques used		67

CHAPTER 4	**ANALYSIS AND INTERPRETATION**	**68-208**

PHASE I - To find out the effect of different dimensions of socio-economic status of family on self-confidence of adolescents. — 68

PHASE II- To find the effect of different dimensions of socio-economic status of family on mental health of adolescents. — 82

PHASE III- To find the effect of different dimensions of socio-economic status of family on personal values of adolescents. — 95

PHASE IV- To see the relationship between self-confidence and mental health of adolescents. — 108

PHASE V- To find the relationship between self- confidence and personal values of adolescents. — 115

PHASE VI- To find the relationship between mental health and personal values of adolescents. — 122

PHASE VII (A)- To find out the effect of locality on the self-confidence of adolescents. — 128

PHASE VII (B)- To find out the effect of locality on the Mental Health of adolescents. — 136

PHASE VII (C)- To find out the effect of locality on the Personal Values of adolescents. — 146

PHASE VIII (A)- To find out the effect of Gender on the Self-Confident of adolescents. — 155

PHASE VIII (B)- To find out the effect of gender on the mental health of adolescents. — 163

PHASE VIII (C)- To find out the effect of gender on the personal values of adolescents. — 173

PHASE IX (A)- To find out the effect of types of school on the self-confidence of adolescents. — 182

PHASE IX (B)- The effect of types of school on Mental Health of adolescents. — 191

PHASE IX (C)- To find out the effect of types of school on the Personal Values of adolescents. — 200

CHAPTER 5	**FINDINGS, CONCLUSION, EDUCAIONAL IMPLICATION AND SUGGESTIONS**	**209-228**
5.1	Main findings	209
5.2	Conclusion	223
5.3	Educational implications	224

5.4	Suggestion	225
	5.4.1. Suggestion for future study	225
	5.4.2 suggestion for parents	226
	5.4.3 suggestion for teacher	227
	5.4.4 suggestion for adolescents	227
	5.4.5 suggestion for policy maker, administrators and educationists	228

CHAPTER-I
INTRODUCTION

INTRODUCTION

Social scientists and sociologists used the term socio-economic status to describe the position of an individual in a society. It includes both social and economic status of an individual in a society. When the socio-economic level of a family is analyzed, household income, level of education, orientation and occupation are analyzed. As well as the combined income and individual characteristic of the household members are also analyzed. **Elizabeth H. baker (2014):** Define socio-economic status as a measure of one's combined economic and social status and it also positively associated with better health. Socio- Economic status is a multidimensional concept and most researchers agree that it includes income of family, education of parents and their occupational status **(Bradly and Crowyn, 2002).** In this study three common elements of socio-economic status, education, income and occupation have been taken. Socio-economic inequalities are an important topic. The socio-economic status of family affects adolescent's lives. Research indicates that SES is an essential factor that affects quality of life of children, youth and families. Family is the first social institution where child is born and brought up by his/her parents and other family members. Family functionality can affect the development and wellbeing of the individual in term of emotionally, mentally and physically. (**Rozumah, Siti Nor, Rojanah and Abdullah al-hadi, 2013; Shak, 2011).**

Low socio- economic status, specifically, is not only a factor but also the causes of many physical and psychosocial stressors. Domestic crowding has been linked to lower SES which is the condition that has negative impact on adults and children, like higher psychological stress and poor health outcomes **(Melki, Beydoun, Khogali, Tamim, &Yunis, 2004).** Low socio-economic status families are suffer from a higher number of stressors related to finances, unemployment and health problems than those with a high socio-economic status **(Senn TE et. al., 2014).** When the socio-economic status of the family is low, the child's up bringing is also affected due to lack of money. The parents are not able to fulfill their needs due to which stress arises in them. **Bradley RH, Corwyn RF, 2002** also revealed that low socio-economic status is connected with high level of stress, poor parenting style and low social environment. Low SES affect adolescent's personality. Many research indicates the relationship between low socio-economic status and Negative psychological health outcomes, **Ikpaya (2004)** found that children who are economically depressed can develop certain psychological feelings which might lead to frustrating performance whereas higher level of SES is related to positive psychological behavior like optimism, self-confidence and well-being. High level of emotional and behavioral difficulties like social problems, delinquent behavior symptoms and lack of attention among adolescents arises due to their low SES **(DeCarlo Santiago, Wadsworth, & Stump, 2011; Russell, Ford, Williams & Russell, 2016; Spencer, Kohn & Woods, 2002).** Low SES produce higher rates of depression, anxiety, suicide attempts, dependency in cigarette and drinking among adolescents **(Newacheck, Hung, Park, Brindis, & Irwin, 2003)** and also produce Higher level of aggression **(Molnar, Cerda, Roberts, & Buka 2008)** and with decreased education success **(Sheridan & Mclaughlin, 2016).** Altogether it can be assumed that low socio-economic status of family is associated stress full life situations, which can increases mental health problems in adolescents.

High socio-economic families give much more importance to education, both with in the household as well as the local community. We know that all educational outcomes of children vary with the SES background of their parents. Family income and parental education can affect student's success. Families with low Socio-economic status have less economic resources to provide academic support to their children. Parents from the low SES groups may be powerless to give these expense of resources such as book, computers or twitters to their children to produce this helpful literacy environment **(Orr, 2003).** Parental education can affect their child's motivation towards learning. Parents with higher SES are in a better position to improve the academic activities of their children as compared to parents with low SES **(Cowen, 2011). Filippin, 2011** found correlation between SES and academic achievement. So we can say that the socio-economic status of family is a factor that determine the academic performance of the adolescents.

In addition to educational outcomes, the socio-economic status of the family also affects the health of the child. **Joseph D.wolfe (2014)** also revealed that Family Income and wealth not only affects early life health, but also affect the health of child and adolescents in different way, children health is affected by their families' wealth, while the health of adolescents is more sensitive to their families' current income. The SES of family affect the physical and mental health of an individual as well as his functions. Children from lower SES families are more likely to have emotional and behavioral problem. This is due to the stress that comes from lack of needed resources such as food, clothes etc. **Sawrey and Telford** opined that children from higher SES are not only brilliant but they also get better opportunities for intellectual, physical and emotional development. **Bandhana and Sharma, Darshan, P. (2010)** found that there are significant differences in mental health of good and poor home environment's secondary students. Children from low socio-economic status families suffer from more health problems than children from high socio-economic status families **(Vukojevic M. et. al., 2017).** In general low income and education are the strong factors affecting physical and mental health problems. **Elgar FJ, Pfortner TK, Moor I, De Clercq B, Stevens GW, Currie C (2015)** also found that adolescents from the families of low SES are more affected by psychological and physical symptoms.

In the personality development of the child, the factor of socio-economic status play an important role. Differences vary in the personality, behavior, mentality etc. of students of different socio-economic level. **Abdur Rahman, ArunavoBairagi, BiplobKumaDey,(2014)** showed that gender and SES have significant effect on adolescents anger, male express more anger than female with low SES than middle and high SES. Also, respondents with middle SES expressed more anger than high SES. Good habits and traditions generate itself in high socio-economic status children. They are well behaved, have good faith and have high level educational achievement and sense of adjustments. But if the situation of the family is contrary to it, then many defects arises in them for example- lacking in adjustments and self-confidence, the emergence of bad habits, inability to make decision etc. It is directly affects their personality. By this the children wander from their path. Family stability and developmental outcomes of children are affected by socio-economic status of family **(Trickett, Aber, Carlson and Cicchetti, 1991).**

Children develop from infancy through adolescence. Adolescence is a term which is derived from the Latin word 'adolescere' which means to 'grow up'. Adolescence is a period of growing up, from the immaturity to maturity. Adolescence is recognized as a period of vital development in which many stresses and strains are experienced by adolescents themselves as well as their parents **(Jersild, 1961).** The adolescent develops with in a complex system of surrounding environment, family, school and cultural values. Adolescence is an important part of human life. Adolescents is a unique developmental period which spreads the gulf between childhood and adulthood **(Smith 2015).**

Adolescents are very sensitive to any changes in their lives. Girls and boys face many physiological and psychological changes in their life. The change in their developmental characteristics bring out change in the parenting role. Parents who is an important component of the family system, plays a significant role in bringing up the children. From this point of view the family is considered as the foundation of the child's development. From the many researches it was found that there is significant effect of parents in shaping the behavior and choice of teens **(Borkowsky, 2002).** Often these changes produce great amounts of stress for them. The level of the stress largely depend upon the nature of the stressors the intelligence level and the coping ability of the individuals **(Soppler, Marks and Adwards, 2012).** Research shows that complex situation in adolescents period, promote so many psychosomatic problem such as anxiety, tension, frustration and emotional upsets. The inability to cope with the changes may lead to other negative consequences such as poor academic performance, low self-confidence and low well- being. Self-confidence is the factor that adolescent emerge from the change in their life.

Self-confidence is a feeling that give rise think in an individual that he or she is capable of doing something with easy way. Self-confidence promote the ability of adjustment, level of happiness and effective functioning in children and adolescents. Self-confidence is one of the qualities of personality that highlights many other qualities in us. It is an important component that shapes the personality of an individual. Self-confidence is not the same in all stage of a person's life. It can be possible that an individual be confident in one area of life and have low confident in some other areas of life. Confidence level can change across the different areas of life. The child's confidence in adolescence sometimes becomes a problem in front of him, because without being confident, the child cannot cope properly with obstacles coming in front of him and become frustrated. According to **Basavanna (1975)** "Self-confidence is the ability of a person to act successfully in an institution to overcome problems and to get things go all right". Many things can influence self-confidence level of a person such as his thoughts, emotions and actions. **Tripathy and Srivastava (2012)** also believed that self-confidence is that attitude by which students believe on their abilities, and they also believed that they can achieve their goals and expectations.

Self-confidence is a mental and spiritual power. Independence of ideas can be gained only by self-confidence. The person who has self-confidence, does not have any kind of worry about his future. It is the internal energy of the person. Self-confidence act as foundation in the development of adolescents. Success and failure of an individual in any work depends on the level of their self-confidence. Without this it is not possible to achieve success in life. People who have high self-confidence are generally happier and more satisfied with their lives than people who have low self-confidence. Other people are easily influenced by the self-confident person and a person's self-confidence control his emotions and behavior.

Two terms mainly related to self-confidence are Self- efficacy and self-esteem. The term self-confidence and self-esteem have been used inter changeably by various psychologists. Self-confidence is major of faith in one's own abilities according to **Cox (2001)** "Self-confidence is a belief in yourself and or abilities, a mental attitude of transiting or relying on yourself" and self-esteem is about our sense of self according to **Rosenberg** Self-esteem is a favorable or unfavorable attitude towards the self . It involves both thoughts and emotions. It is believed that a person who have high level of self- esteem will may be confident. Similarly, if a person has a negative self-view, which can cause them to lack of confidence in many situations, particularly in tasks that involve problem solving skill. A relationship has also been found between self-esteem and anxiety level many researchers found that an increase in self-esteem result in a decline of internal and reactive anxiety and vice versa **(Erol and Orth, 2011; Riaz and Sarwat, 2013; Lee and Hankin, 2009).**

Self-confidence is an important role in adolescence, because adolescence is a state of life where the child encounters many problems. In this stage adolescents get very excited. In such situation it is necessary to have confidence in them so that they can identify themselves and choose the correct path. **(Sears, Albert 1990).** According to **Ceibb (2003)** "Self-confidence is the result of a successfully handle risk". As one who has a high self-confidence tends to have a stable mind and express himself or herself, it can be assumed that he or she is likely to have a good mental health compared with the one has a low self- confidence. Because when child have confidence then he take such decision that are good for him and his health. Self-Confidence can also give him a positive outlook on life which can increase his mental and emotional well-being. However, when he lacks of self-confidence, his self-esteem can also be affected and that starts affecting his health as well. When a child lacks self-confidence, it becomes difficult for him to make the right decision and face challenges. He starts doubting himself. He found it difficult to face the crowd and he starts avoiding many situations. Which can give rise to negativity in him.

The child's confidence influence his academic achievement. **Lal. K. (2014)** found a significant relationship between academic achievement and self-confidence of male and female adolescents. **Dhall S. Thukral P (2013)** revealed that there is a significant and positive relationship between intelligence and self-confidence and also between intelligence and academic achievements of a child. So it can be say that self-confidence is an important factor for adolescent's achievement. Most of the problems in the education system is arises due to student's low self-confidence that lead a number of students having lack of enough participation and unsatisfactory progress **(Norman aHyland 2003).** Self-confidence is very necessary for a students to take participation in the learning activities, those who have self-confidence they have a belief on their abilities and they set goals and work hard to achieve them without worrying about the outcomes **(Kanza, 2016). Verma and Kumari, (2016); Singh, Y.G., (2010)** also found that there is a relation between self-confidence and academic achievement. Rather than achievement Self-confidence is reported to have a significant impact on life outcomes for e.g. self-confidence and adjustment **(Kumar, 2003)** self-confidence and problem solving ability **(Srimadevi and Sarladevi, 2016)** self-confidence and intelligence **(Dhall, S., Thukral, P., 2013).** Like self-confidence, in the development of mental disorders and social problems such as depression, anxiety and violence, there is a role of self-esteem as well. **(Mann et. al., 2004).** Low self-confidence is related to different dimension of stress such as academic stress, inter personal stress, environmental stress etc. **(Salvaraj and Ganadevan, 2014).** Factors such as gender socio-economic status, personality and mental health and support from family are all have an important effect on the self-confidence of adolescents.

Along with self-confidence, mental health and personal values in adolescence also affect the development of the teenager. Mental health is a way that describe social and emotional well-being. According to WHO " mental health is a state of well-being in which every individual realizes his or her own potential, can cope with the normal stresses of life can work productively and fruitfully and is able of make a contribution to his or her community". Mental health of an individual states that how he look at himself, his lives, and the other people in his lives and can evaluate his challenges and problems effectively. This includes how to handle stress, how to relate with other people, and how to take decisions **(Panchal, 2013).** Mental Health is the ability to balance emotions, desires, ambitions and ideals one's daily life. It means that it is ability to face and accept the realities of life **(Bhatia, 1984).**

Mental health is associated with the adjustment and socially acceptable behavior. It is the ability of a person which helps him to face and accept the reality of life. According to **A.K. Menninger** "mental health is the ability of adjustment of a person to the world and to each other with a maximum of effectiveness and happiness". It is the ability to manage an even temper, an alert intelligence, socially acceptable behavior and a happy disposition". A mentally healthy person is well adjusted to social rules, he accept the reality of life and has minimum tension. Mental health is such a condition as well as a level of function which is accepted socially and satisfied personally **(Mudasir 2013).** The main characteristic of mental health, is adjustment, higher the adjustment level of a person, the greater will be the mental health of individual and if the mental health of a person is low than his adjustment level will also be low. Good mental health provide positive feelings and attitudes towards the self and towards the other. **Srividhya, V.; and Khadi, Puspha, B (2007)** found a relation between mental health and adjustment problems which indicates that higher adjustment problems related with low the mental health.

Mental health is a condition of emotional stability. Emotional stability is that ability which help a person to cope with general change in the environment. The emotional stability may be related with peace of mind and may be free from anxiety and stress **(Hay and Ashman 2003).** The emotional balance is disturbed in adolescence. This is the period of intensive stress and strain. They are two sensitive, inflammable and moody. Low self-confidence, anxiety, depression, adjustment problem, lack of interest etc. are some of the emotional problems observed in the adolescents subjected to dysfunctional parenting.

Poor mental health may be effects the wider health and development of adolescents and due to this some bad habits like drinking alcohol, eating tobacco, school dropout and delinquent behavior may be arise in the adolescents. Adolescence is considered a stage of problems. Adolescents have adjustment problems. This problem creates frustration in them which affects their whole personality. A mentally healthy person is able to adjust properly with his environment. Generally mental health is reflected in symptoms like anxiety, tension restlessness or hopelessness among others **(Pooja, et. al. 2012).** Adjustment of adolescents at home and at school is a burning issue of the present time. They are now found suffering from mental illness, drug addiction in great number, alcoholism. Suicides and crimes have become common among adolescents, psychological disorder and SES of family may be the root of these problems. According to the family stress model economic hardship negatively affects children's psychological adjustment indirectly through its effects on the parent's behavior toward the child **(V.C. Mcloyd et. al., 2009)**.

Adolescents experience stress in their life. Long term exposal to stress is associated with many psychological and physiological illness in addition to smoking, drug abuse and sexual behavior **(Aggarwal S. 2007)**. Academic stress is an important factor of stress among adolescents and it may decrease self-confidence of adolescents. **Chaing (1995)** purposed that school is one of the main source of stress among adolescents, this stress come from too much homework, preparation for test, lack of interest in particular subject and punishment given by the teacher. Self-confidence and problem solving skill can help to prevent mental health problems such as anxiety, depression etc. An anxiety and stress, lack of confidence lead to depression, anger and other mental health problems. **Rosenberg M. et. al., (1995)** found that self-esteem is associated with depression and anxiety.

Adolescents are the future citizens of a nation. They act as a resources for the nation. Adolescence period is associated with the cognitive, emotional and attitudinal change characteristics of adolescents and wrong change in them can cause stress and depression among adolescents. The most common problems in adolescence is depression **(Kessler et. al., 2001; Pennant et al., 2015)**. Moreover, depression give rise to negative results like academic difficulties, interpersonal dysfunction and health problems **(Berndt et. al., 2000; Zlotnick et. al., 2000)**. Many prior studies have been found that family context and internal resources are an important factors that are associated with adolescent's depression **(Elovainio et. al., 2012; Sichko et. al., 2015)**. In the family context Socio-economic status and parenting are two important basic factors which affect the development of adolescents. The link between socio-economic status of family and adolescents depression has been found. The mental health of adolescents is also affected by the parent's income and education. **Glasscock DJ. et. al., (2013)** also found that low parental income and education were associated with high level of stress regardless of adolescent's gender. Therefore, parental income, education and occupation may be linked with adolescents' depression.

Self-confidence and personal values are the two main characteristics of positive mental health. Personal Values of an individual are those characteristics and behavior that motivate him to do right work and guide him to take right decisions. Personal Value of an individual are a reflection of his highest principle of mind and thought and it can be said to part of spiritual domain. There are the guiding principles of life, which lead to all round development of an individual **Allport (1961)** defines it as "A belief on which a man act by preference". Personal values determine the uniqueness of an individual and most of it gets developed in us even unconsciously during experiencing some difficult periods in our life. Personal values are associated with the choice of an individual. We take decisions and choose behaviors, friends, jobs and hobbies according to our personal values **(Verma and Panwar)**. Values can be considered as the ultimate development of those many process of selection and generalization that produce long range consistency and organization in individuals **(Converse 1965)**.

Values are important for one's personality development. Values play an important role in living life successfully. Values are reflected in the way a person behave, talks and understands. It help a person to achieve the academic and professional excellence which make them a good citizen of the country. It is not only helps one to differentiate between good and bad but also helps one to handle difficult situation systematically. A person develops his values directly through parents at home and the teachers at school and then from society. These may also be obtained from those particular groups or systems like cultures, religion etc. **Blais (2010)** suggested that personal values can be developed by family, culture, society, environment, religious believe and ethnicity. **Natasha (2013)** reported that adolescents from urban and rural areas give first preference to social values because both are resourceful and they can develop traits like love, sympathy and kindness into their behaviour. They give second preference to political values. So we can say that personal values are not universal. The nature of family, nation and society affects personal values of an individual. A person's personal values help him to differentiate between good and bad, beneficial and harmful, important and not important, useful and useless, desirable and unwanted etc. so personal values are those view point, philosophy, ideology that are significant in the person life.

Home is the first school of the child where his socialization takes plays. The family teach the child the cultural and traditional values. **Robert REL, Bengtson VL. (1999),** stated that families are an important factor for the development of children's values. The child does not learn only good behavior but he also learn social and moral values. Values are beliefs or ideals shared by the member of society which tell about what is good or bad and right or wrong. Values influence the person's behavior and attitude and gives suitable guidelines in all situations. When particular values are strong and silent to individuals, they are generally motivated to behave in ways that one consistent with their goals **(Boyce et. al., 2013)**.

Adolescence is that stage of development during which personal values develops **(Daniel et al., 2012)**. Personal values are transmitted to children from their parents. **(Benish- Weisman et. al., 2017)**. But in adolescence period, adolescents are more influenced by their peers then by parents **(Benish- Weisman et. al., 2017)**. That is why the values transferred by the parents start changing in adolescents. Personal values mainly affect the behavior of adolescents. **Kasai, K., Fukuda M., (2017)** stated that personal values is a broad goal which varying according to the person's importance, guiding attitudes and behavior. Personal values are those values which influence person's behavior and by which an individual is committed **(Theodorson and Achilles, 1969)**. These are most important factor to determine the personality of every adolescents. Personal values are our believes on honesty, love, helpfulness, courage, discipline, good manners, cleanliness and faithfulness. They influence person's action and reaction. Person make decisions on the basis of their personal values and also choose their behavior, friends, employment and entertainment in large part on their personal values. In this research, the personal values of adolescents has been investigated on the bias of the following dimensions.

1. **Honesty** –Honesty refers to a facet of moral character and denotes positive, virtuous attributes such as integrity, truthfulness and straightforwardness along with absence of lying, cheating and theft.
2. **Love-** A sense of regard and affection based on admiration towards any person.
3. **Helpfulness-** The property of providing useful assistance, friendliness evidence by a kindly disposition.
4. **Courage-** A quality of moral and mental spirit that enables you to face danger, a position or pain without showing fear.
5. **Good manners-** The correct way of acting etiquette, being courteous and polite to others. Faithfulness the quality of being loyal and doing the right thing for the right person's.
6. **Discipline-** A systematic method of obtaining obedience, self-control, remove bad habits and set of rules regulating behaviors in the right way.
7. **Cleanliness-** Good hygiene, neatness of person.

There are various types of values such as moral values, family values, social cultural values, material values, spiritual values, personal values, etc. Personal values are those principle on his we build our life. They are the combination of family values and social cultural values. Our personal values help us to think about what is good for us (e.g. honesty, love, faithfulness, discipline etc.). Different people have different values. A particular values may be important for one person but may be unimportant for another person. Therefore an individual's personal values are unique. No two individuals, have alike personal values.

Like self-confidence and mental health, personal values is also influenced by the SES of the family. **Nagrajan Pavithra, Ahuja Abha and Singh Ritu (2020)** revealed that the family income of family plays an important role in the personal values of adolescents. The education of parents affects the personal values of the child. Educated parents teach children to identify right and wrong. In adolescence, children are ready to cross the limit of aggression. In such situation their personal values show them the right path. Child's personal values also affect his mental health. **Yasuma N., Watanable K, Lida M, Nishi D, Kawakami N, (2019)** revealed that in during active challenging, cherishing family and friends and the commitment to values were significantly and negatively associated with psychological distress in adults. According to **Vasuki (2003)** gender, locality, type and system of school affects the values of the students. **Susan and Anupama (1998)** found that high academic achievers had higher values than the low achievers and **Manivannan (2003)** revealed that gender did not have an impact on the attitudes of students towards values.

Adolescence is the period of life when the surge of life reaches its highest peak. Adolescents with the high self-confidence, good mental health and personal values are considered to achieve their identity in the society, develop leadership qualities, whereas lake of these qualities lead to frustration, stress, rejection and discouragement. In adolescence period for the development of adolescent self-confidence, mental health and personal values play an important role. Along with family environment, socio-economic status of the family also play an important role in the development of self-confidence, mental health and personal values of adolescents.

1.1 ORIGIN OF THE STUDY

Adolescence is such a state of life, when different fluctuations in the life of child occurs. At this period, adolescents have to face many problems. To cope with these problems it is necessary to have self-confidence, good mental health and personal values in them. Self-confident person is free from all types of internal conflicts. He formally cope up with all kinds of difficulties. **According to Bandura (1986),** "self-confidence is considered one of the most influential motivators and regulators of behavior in people's everyday lives". Possessing self-confidence, mental health and personal values a person can adjust himself properly in his environment and make the best efforts for the progress and betterment of his family and society. Many changes in adolescence affect the adjustment level, their beliefs and behavior of adolescents. It is necessary to give positive direction to these effects so that qualities of self-confidence, personal values etc. can be developed.

During adolescence there are changes in the personality of the adolescent, in his mental health and personal values. He has to make his identity in the society. The development of the personality of an adolescents in a positive direction is beneficial for the society and the country. The socio-economic status of the family can influence the personality development of the adolescent. Where on one hand the socio-economic status of the family provides the right direction to his personality, on the other hand it also has a negative effect on it. Parents are responsible for giving the right direction to personality development of and adolescents. **Nagiach, 1987** also stated that parenting style had a great influence on a personality development and disposition of the children. Parent's education and occupation effect adolescents in different way. His achievement, his decision making power, emotional maturity, self-confidence values all depends on his parenting style. Educated parents teach the child to recognize right and wrong. Instills confidence in them. Teach the child to adjust with the environment and also teach him to corporate with other live with love.

The period of adolescence is the more difficult period in the human development. During this period a person confronts with growing severe difficulties and manifests conditions symptomatic of great emotional tensions, which create mental disorders. Adolescents wants to feel and act grown up. In many instances however the adolescent's lack of confidence and self-assurance makes it very difficult for them to satisfactorily accomplish this objective. Self-confident people believe in their abilities, capacities and judgment. A feeling of self-confidence can help an individual to feel better and help him to over-come difficulties. As a result, they do not have any kind of panic while facing any new and unfamiliar situation.

The thing which has more demand in all the societies of the world, is the need to keep up mental health of the individual. A person's behavior is determine by his physical and mental factors. Mental health is an important factor that helps in the maintenance of physical health as well as social adjustment. The mental health of the person affects his personal values and self-confidence. It is commonly seen that if the mental health is good then the ideal values and confidence will arise in the persons because a mentally healthy person evaluates himself properly. A mentally healthy person may be aware from his own tendencies by observing himself so that he can divert them in the right directions. He has own ideas, thoughts and opinion, he is a cool person who deals calmly with every circumstances, without fear, disturbance, anxiety and stress. **Neelima, M. (2013)** found a positive correlation between self-confidence and mental health. Positive thinking is beneficial for mental and emotional well-being and it also boost self-confidence. A mentally healthy person have a desirable attitudes, healthy values and right self-concept and a scientific perception of the world. Several Psychologists like **Rogers (1961), Hurlock (1972) and Erickson (1936)** have also given similar views.

Family and school can play an important role in the development of self-confidence, mental health and personal values of adolescents. Early in life the family has an impact on the child's mental health and personal values, but in adolescence these are more influenced by the school environment, peer group and community. We feel that the socio- economic status of the family along with family environment may also affects the child's self-confidence, mental health and personal values. Socio-economic status include education, occupation and income of family. Parent's high educational level may create high values in children on the other hand if the family income is low, then they may not fulfill the needs of the children which may lead to conflict in them arise and their mental health decrease. The proper fulfillment of the requirements of the adolescents by their parents make them become optimistic and altruistic. But when parents don't fulfill their requirements they become pessimistic and selfish. Family environment, behavior of parents, poverty, discipline of home, family stress etc. are some factors that affect the mental health of adolescents. But on the other side we also see that even if parents are not educated, they put high values in their children and even when the family income is low there is a lot of confidence and high mental health in the adolescents.

Socio-economic status of the family has a great influence on the personality development and the disposition of the adolescents. Researcher feel that it would not be wrong to say that socio- economic status of family guides an individual to become more confident, mentally healthy and personally valued. For the unique and dynamic personality self-confidence, mental health and personal values are must. Thus all the four factors i.e. socio economic status, self-confidence, mental health and personal values may be interlinked with each other and adolescence being the transition period seen to be most affected one with all the four. Thus efforts should be made to enhance the self-confidence, mental health and personal values of the adolescents. Thus the purpose of the investigation is **"A study of impact of socio- economic status on self-confidence, mental health and personal values of adolescents".**

1.2 SIGNIFICANCE OF THE STUDY

In this research, student of senior secondary level have been taken as adolescents. At this stage the adolescents have made their identity in the society. He moves towards his goal. In this stage, he need the help of his parents and teachers. They guide them to make their identity in the society. Adolescence is the peak period of growth and development that occurs between childhood and adult hood. The overall development of adolescents who are the future nation builders is a very vital and cardinal question .The balanced development of adolescents is essential not only for parent's satisfaction and happiness but also for growth and advancement of any nation. Adolescents are more demanding and harder in these days than even before .They are also very disappointed and frustrated, hence defiant and disobedient .High level of frustration leads to drug addiction etc. which became harmful for youth as well as society. Today it is a burning problem in which solution is essential **(Sharma and Sinha 2004).**

This is the age when an adolescents has to make his identity in the society. Sometimes their scholastic performance may not be good enough to make his identity in the society. And not being able to make his identity in the society, can create tension in him. Adolescent's confidence and mental health may be helpful in reliving this stress. Because **Basavanna (1975),** define Self-confidence as an ability of a person to act effectively and to overcome obstacles and to get things go all right. According to **A.K. Menninger** "mental health is the ability of adjustment of a person with world and to each other with more of effectiveness and happiness". It is the ability which maintain an individual's temper, intelligence, socially acceptable behavior and happy disposition.

The self-confidence and mental health of a person gives him the courage to tackle any problem. At this modern era to increase the spirit of brother hood among the individuals, good personal values also need to be highlighted among them.

Adolescence have to face some physical and mental problems. They also have the problem of adjustment. It is very critical period in the life of an adolescence. If he does not get the right guidance at this time, then many mental complication may arise in him. In adolescence, there is a rapid change in personality, in the goal of living and in attitude towards self and other people. Industrialization in India has brought about many social changes. As a result, adolescence have to get higher education and training to get job. At the same time, due to industrialization the competition has increased so much that it is not possible for everyone to get a good job. Adolescence is an age where adolescents are concerned about their career and if for some reason he is not able to reach his goal, then his self-confidence starts following. This creates tension in him which can affects his personal values as well.

Self-confidence, mental health and personal values mainly affects the behavior of adolescents. These are developed and influenced by the home environment. Home environment affected by the socio economic status of the family and facilities available in the home. Therefore the socio-economic status of the family may also effect the self-confidence, mental health and personal values of adolescents. If the self-confidence, mental health and personal values are not developed in adolescents they will not live their life easily, then it may rise to many behavior related problems. In the absence of these characteristics the growth of a person in a social and professional life may effected. Adolescents who have poor self-confidence, mental health and personal values cannot fit into a normal situation. Thus they become a problem not only for themselves but also for home, school and society. A confident person has the power to face any situation fearlessly. In the present time Self-confidence has become a most common characteristics. Teachers, parents and others all give their focus on boosting the self-confidence of child. People, high in self-confidence are attractive and to make better impression on other's than people with low self-confidence. A mentally healthy person adjust easily to his environment. He is emotionally stable. He free from fear, apprehension or anxiety, tension etc. and he has such a mental ability which helps him to think reasonably and in acting purposefully in his environment. While the dimension of personal values are honesty, love, courage, helpfulness, good manners, faithfulness, discipline and cleanliness.

Family is the first school of child development because the etiquettes received from the family makes strong character of children as they play an important role in making an ethical citizen by giving them the right direction. In a country like India, it is often found that all the needs of the child are met by the family. The level of the fulfillments influences his self-confidence, mental health and personal values, which have a tendency to make an identity and expression of thoughts and action in adolescents. In the absence of such a motivation adolescents becomes frustrated and their life gets complicated than ever before. In today's modern environment, if an adolescents cannot adjust himself then he becomes frustrated which generates many bad habits in him. So the researcher feels that, in order to overcome all these problems, adolescents may develop self-confidence, good mental health and ideal personal values in them.

Along with the family environment the socio and economic status of the family may also have a greater influence in the development of the adolescents. The income, education and occupation of the parents constitute the socio-economic status of family, that could be considered as a developmental factor of self-confidence, mental health and personal values in individuals at various stage of development. The socioeconomic status of the family may affect the self-confidence, mental health and personal values of adolescents. Therefore the researcher feels that the socio-economic status of family may help to improve the self-confidence, mental health and personal values of adolescents. There is a need to develop the self-confidence, mental health and personal values in adolescents. Better self-confidence, mental health and personal values may serve as a helping hand for problem solving, better productivity, good quality of life and improved performance. Therefore the researcher feels that for all round development of adolescents all these factors (Self-confidence, Mental health and Personal values) are required. So it is necessary to develop the self-confidence, mental health and personal values of an adolescents. Moreover, it is quite evident that self-confidence, mental health and personal values may be interlinked with each other.

In the development of a child the role of school is very important after home. Because the child spends most of the time in school. School is the place where child face many problems. Therefore, it is the responsibility of teacher to make every effort to make his classroom healthy for the development of the child. It is the responsibility of the school to inculcate self-confidence and good values in child. At the same time school should provide such environment to the children so that they remain mentally and physically healthy. Now there is a need to reform education system to increase self-confidence in the learners, remove mental stress and develop good personal values. These means that such programs should be included in the curriculum which can develop the child in the right direction.

Adolescence is a very important stage of life having lot of enthusiasm, energy an aspiration, which can be channelized in good direction by their parents and teachers **(Sharma and Sinha, 2004).** Family, school and media have become very important for the proper development of the adolescence. In this era of industrialization, the socio-economic status of families has varied. Which has created a situation of tension in the families. **Mathur and Pareek (2003)** reported that rapid change in society and complexities around them affect adolescent's psychological development. Suicides and crimes have become so common among adolescents, the prevention of these problems is essential not only at individual and community level, but it must be taken care of globally. On the other hand, when the parents provide love and support to the children and give them the power to solve the problems with confidents, then there is not any kind of mental disorder rises in the adolescence. The concept of self-confidence, mental health and personal values are an emerging field of research in the area of social, behavior and management science. The researcher feels that for the harmonious and all round development of an adolescents, balanced and healthy environment is also required.

In many researches, the impact of the socio-economic status of the family has been seen in various aspects of the child development. The study of many researches reveals that a lot of studies have been made on SES, self-confidence, mental health or personal values separately. But no study or only few studies have been conducted taking the impact of SES of the family on self-confidence, mental health and personal values of adolescents into considerations. It is also justified that whatever studies have been made previously do not employee hair due to demographic characteristics and cultural difference. This explains the importance of the present study to investigate the effect of socio-economics status on the self-confidence, mental health and personal values of adolescents in the present situation.

The finding of the study will be useful for teacher, parents, institution in doing their respective job. The result of this study will help to overcome the problems of gender difference, region and socio-economic status which influence the self-confidence, mental health and personal values of adolescents. Policymakers can minimize the problem of adolescents related to gender difference and socio-economic status which cause low self-confidence, mental health and personal values, by conducting seminars and workshop, which enhance the self-confidence, mental health and personal values of adolescents.

1.3 STATEMENT OF THE PROBLEM

The present investigation is undertaken **"TO STUDY THE IMPACT OF SOCIO-ECONOMIC STATUS OF FAMILY ON SELF-CONFIDENCE, MENTAL HEALTH AND PERSONAL VALUES OF ADOLESCENTS"**

1.4 DELIMITATIONS

In order to concretize the problem, following controls have been applied.

(1) This study were conducted in Intermediate schools of Dehradun District only.

(2) Both male and female students studying in class 11th and 12thvof government, government aided recognized by Uttarkhand Board, and non-government intermediate schools situated in Urban and rural areas of Dehradun District were included in survey.

(3) The rural area is not extreme rural but peri-urban/ sub-urban area as it is situated close to the urban area.

1.5 FUNCTIONAL AND OPERATIONAL DEFINITION OF THE KEY TERMS

1.5.1 SOCIO-ECONOMIC STATUS

"Socio-economic Status (SES) is the term used to distinguish between people's relative position in the society in terms of family income, political power, educational background and occupational prestige".

Parson et al. (2001)

OPERATIONAL DEFINITION- In the present study, parent's education, income and occupation constitute the socio-economic status of family. The socio-economic status of adolescents' family has been determined by the Modified Kuppuswamy scale (2018).

1.5.2 SELF-CONFIDENCE

"Self-confidence refers to an individual's perceived ability to act effectively in an institution to overcome obstacles and to get things go all right".

Basavanna (1975)

"Self-confidence is considered one of the most influential motivator and regulators of behavior in people's everyday lives"

Bandura (1986)

OPERATIONAL DEFINITION- In the present study the meaning of self-confidence is the ability of adolescents to express themselves and the ability to face any circumstances boldly. This has been taken as mean self-confidence score obtained on Dr. Rekha Gupta, self-confidence inventory.

1.5.3 MENTAL HEALTH

Mental health is " a state of well –being in which the individual realizes his or her own abilities, can cope with the normal stresses of life, can work productively and fruitfully, and is able to make a contribution to his or her community."

According to WHO

"Let us define mental health as the adjustment of human being to the world and to each other with a maximum of effectiveness and happiness. It is the ability to maintain an ever temper, an alert intelligence, socially considerate behavior and happy disposition."

A.K. Menninger

OPERATIONAL DEFINITION- Here mental health refers to the adolescent's adjustment, emotional stability, autonomy, security-insecurity, self-concept and intelligence. This has been taken as mean mental health score obtained on **Arun Kumar Sing and Alpana Sen Gupta,** mental health battery.

1.5.4 PERSONAL VALUES

"Personal values or individual values are the values to which an individual is committed and which influences his behavior".

Theodorson and Achilles, 1969

OPERATIONAL DEFINITION- In the present study personal values refers to the characteristics of adolescents as honesty, love, helpfulness, courage, good manners, discipline and cleanliness. In the present study personal values is a measure on the scale of the Personal Value scale by Dr. Madhulika Verma.

1.5.5 ADOLESCENT

"Adolescents can be defined as a stage in the life cycle between 13 and 18 years of age characterized by increasing independence from adult controls, rapidly occurring physical and psychological change, exploration of social issues and concerns increased focus on activities with a peer group and establishment of a basic self- identity"

Bigner (1983)

"Sociologically, adolescence is the transition period from depended childhood to self-sufficient adult hood. Psychologically, it is a "Marginal situation" in which new adjustment have to be made, namely those that distinguished child behavior from adult behavior in a given society. Chronologically, it is the time span from approximately twelve or thirteen to the early twenties with wide individual and cultural variations."

Muuss (1962)

OPERATIONAL DEFINITION- In the present study students studying in 11th and 12th has been considered as adolescents.

1.6 OBJECTIVES OF THE STUDY

The present study aims at accomplishing the following objectives:

1. To find out the effect of different dimensions of socio-economic status of family on self-confidence of adolescents.

2. To find the effect of different dimensions of socio-economic status of family on mental health of adolescents.
3. To find the effect of different dimensions of socio-economic status of family on personal values of adolescents.
4. To find out the relationship between self-confidence and mental health of adolescents.
5. To find out the relationship between self-confidence and personal values of adolescents.
6. To find out the relationship between mental health and personal values of adolescents.
7. To find out the effect of locality on self-confidence, mental health and personal values of adolescents.
8. To compare self-confidence, mental health and personal values of adolescent on the basis of gender differences.
9. To find out the effect of types of school on self-confidence, mental health, and personal values of adolescents.

CHAPTER-II
REVIEW OF LITERATURE

REVIEW OF RELATED LITERATURE

Review of Literature has two words- 'Literature' and 'Review'. The term literature is traditional used to refer to language. But in the field of research, the term literature refers to the knowledge of a particular area of research of a subject while the meaning of the term review into arrange the knowledge of a particular area of research and expand the knowledge to see that the study done by him will be a contribution in this field.

Generally every type of information contained in written or Verbal, Printed or handwritten, books or journals etc., which is connected to research problem, is known as Review of related literature.

Every research starts from where previous research has left it. Therefore, it is very important for every researcher to be well aware of the information of literature related to their problem, done by others. It is considered extremely important in actual planning and study.

Related Literature helps the researcher to define his/her problem. On this basis, the researcher makes his hypothesis. The review of literature suggests the researcher for appropriate method, procedure and statical techniques to solve the problem. Therefore, literature review has a very important place in the success of any research.

Keeping the above information in mind, this chapter present a brief review of previously conducted researches related to socio-economic status, adolescent's self-confidence, mental health and personal values. For the convenience of the investigator, this chapter is broadly divided into four parts.

1. Studies on Socio-economic Status
2. Studies on Self Confidence.
3. Studies on Mental Health
4. Studies on Personal Values.

2.1 STUDIES ON SOCIO-ECONOMIC STATUS

According to **Trickett, Aber, Carlson, &Cicchetti, 1991,** Socioeconomic status affects family stability which includes parenting practices and developmental outcomes for children. Socio-economic status affects various aspect of adolescents like his health, self-confidence, mental health, personal values, achievement etc. All these aspect of adolescents cannot be adequately researched in a single study. Therefore the investigator intended to study the socio-economic status under following broad heading.

1. Socio-economic status and health
2. Socio-economic status and achievement
3. Socio-economic status and self-confidence
4. Socio-economic status and mental health
5. Socio-economic status and personal values

2.1.1 SOCIO-ECONOMIC STATUS AND HEALTH

The socio-economic level of the family consist the income, education and occupation of parents. Due to lack of money in families with low SES the child is not able to be brought up properly, which affects his health. According to **Elizabeth H. baker (2014),** Socio-economic status is a measure of one's combined economic and social status and it is positively associated with better health. **Bradly and Crowyn, (2002),** said that Socio- Economic status is a multidimensional concept and most researchers agree that it is represented by a combination of family income, parental education and occupational status. **Joseph D. Wolfe (2014)** revealed that family income and wealth not only affects early life health but also affects child and adolescent health in a different way. Children's health is more sensitive to the wealth of their families, while adolescents' health is more sensitive to the current income of their families. Together, the neutralizing effects of family income and wealth negate one another such that the overall effect of economic conditions on health is the same for children and adolescents. **Bradley and Corwyn (2002)** have reviewed a large number of studies on the effects of SES on children's development, particularly over health, cognitive and academic attainment, and socio emotional development. Regarding the relationship between SES and health, they found that low-SES children and adolescents are more likely to have several health problems. These health problems include growth retardation, birth defects, fetal alcohol syndrome, depression, obesity, and stunting during the teenage years.

Senn TE, Walsh JL, Carey MP. (2014) and Weyers S, Dragano N, Mobus S, Beck EM, Stang A, Mohlenkamp S (2010) found that families with a low socioeconomic status (SES) are deprived in multiple ways and suffer from a number of stressors related to finances, social relationship, employment and health problems as compared to high SES families. **Vukojevic M, Zovko A, Talic I, Tanovic M, Resic**

B, Vrdoljak I (2017) also found that children with low SES suffer more often from health problems than children with high SES. Further **Sawrey and Telford** revealed that children from higher SES are not only brilliant but they also have more opportunities for intellectual, physical and emotional development. **Pascoe JM, Wood DL, Duffee JH, Akno A, et.al., 2016; Chaudhary A, Wimer, C 2016; Racine AD, 2016,** also found that the children of families living in poverty are more likely to have health conditions and poorer health status, as well as lower access to and use of health care services.

Dmitrieva (2013) places socioeconomic status (SES) in the context of the psychology of adolescent development. It is particularly useful to observe the mechanisms mediating the association between SES and health in adolescence, such as access to resources, psychosocial mechanisms (stress, emotional processing, health behaviors, and exposure to risky social environments), and biological mechanisms. **Inchley, et al. (2016)** presents survey findings from 42 countries on SES (as indicated by a measure of family affluence) differences in subjective health, self-reported health behaviours, and psychosocial environment. The report revealed that, in general, young people in countries and regions with large differences in wealth distribution are more sensitive to poorer health outcomes and independent of their individual family wealth. **Quon and McGrath (2014)** reports on the association between socio-economic status (SES) and health outcomes during adolescence, demonstrating that socio-economic status is associated with health during adolescence. Similarly **Okamota, S.(2021)** revealed that parents socio-economic status associated with child health related outcomes. **Chen, Matthews, & Boyce, 2002; and Pamuk, Makuc, Heck, Reuben, & Locher, 1998** revealed that Low socio-economic status has a profound influence on physical health throughout childhood. **Pamuk et al., 1998** further revealed that children lower in socio-economic status have higher rate of many diseases, including higher blood pressure, lower rate of physical activities, and greater likelihood of smoking. **Evans & English, 2002 and Sandberg et al., 2000,** found that stressful life circumstances, have been linked to negative biological and health outcomes in children.

2.1.2 SOCIO-ECONOMIC STATUS AND ACHIEVEMENT

Parental education have a significant role on their child's motivation towards learning. **Cowen, (2011)** revealed that parents from high SES are in a better position to improve the academic performance of their children as compared to parents from low SES. According to **Denga (1986)** home environment to a great extent, affects the child's behaviour and achievement. He also said that home conditions like noise, poor accommodation, poor lightening for reading and lack of educational materials have negative effect on the child's learning ability. He went on to suggest that for effectiveness and success in learning, there must be adequate reading space and a challenging environment for the child. Further **Sharma and Tahira (2011)** found That Parent's Education had a Significant Relation with Children Achievement. **Sheridan & Mclaughlin, (2016)** also found that lower level of SES are associated with decreased education success. **Felner et. al., (1995)** reported that the youth whose parents were employed in low income, unskilled occupation were found to have lower level of school performance compared to those where adults were in high paying occupation. Adolescents from families in which parents had not graduated from high school presented significantly poor socio-emotional and academic adjustment. The sources further explained that these children did not only have a smaller vocabulary than children from more healthy areas (upper class) but their words had some special meaning in their dialect. **Orr, (2003)** revealed that parents from the low SES groups may be powerless to meet the expense of resources such as book, computers or twitters to produce this helpful literacy environment.

Borbora, Rupa Das (1998) carried out a study on the impact of socioeconomic status on the academic achievement of the first generation learner. A positive and significant relationship between SES and Academic Achievement was found in a study conducted by **Faaz and Khan (2017)** on Academic Achievement of upper primary school students in relation to their Socio-economic Status. **Md Rofikul Islam and ZebunNisa Khan (2017)** found is positive correlation between Socio-economic Status and Academic Achievement of Senior Secondary School students. It also presented a significant difference among different SES group in their Academic Achievement. They also revealed that there is no significant difference between the academic achievement of male and female students. On the other side **Gupta and Katoch (2013) & Debrah, K., (2018)** revealed that there was no significant relationship between SES and Academic Achievement. **Sukhwant Bajwa and Shalu Jindail (2005)** of Punjab University took up a study on under achievement in science in relation to intelligence and socio-economic status. The sample consisted of 2000 students of class 11th randomly taken from three schools of Chandigarh. The result showed a significant difference in high intelligent and low intelligent on variable of under achievement. There was significant difference between high socio-economic status and low economic status on the variable of under achievement. No Interaction effect of socio-economic status and intelligence on under achievement in science was found and the result showed that the five variables compositely predicted academic performance of students. They also revealed that the resident factor rather than other factor in the child uniquely predicted academic performance of the respondent. Further **Pradhan, Dibyaprava (1997)** carried out a study to see the effect of socioeconomic status and intelligence on scholastic achievement of girls. He was found that SES is not effective with regard to scholastic achievement. Intelligence is significantly and positively associated with self-confidence and socio-economic status **(Dhall and Thukral, 2009 and Al-Hebaish, 2012). Ebong (2004), Tina (2001) Mgbado (2002)** revealed that the socio-economic status of parents play an important role in the retention of students in not only Social Studies but in school subjects generally. They further reported that the best simple predictor of the child's future achievement is the family status.

Showkeen and Rehman (2014) conducted a study about the effects of Socio-economic Status of Science stream students and their Academic Achievement at Senior Secondary level. The study showed significant and positive relationship between SES and Academic performance of Science stream students of Senior Secondary level. **Prabha and Gupta, Monika (2000)** made an attempt to find out of the effect of sex, intelligence and socio-economic status on the achievement of student in computer education. In the sample all the students of calls 11th who were studying computer as a subject were selected form five convent schools in Agra City. Data was collected through various tools- Group intelligence tests, SES scale and marks secured by students in the computer examination. The important result is that is that there is significant relationship between SES and computer achievement. Further **Rather and Sharma (2015)** conducted a study on the effects of Socio-economic Status on Achievement grades. They found that there was a close relationship between SES and Academic grades of the students. They also revealed that rather than female student male students performs better and got better marks. They further showed that there was no significant difference between the academic performance of urban and rural students. **Mahmood, Ali (1998)** conducted a study to develop a view of prediction about the students on the basis of their personal values, career ambitions, socio-economic status and academic achievement. He found that the academic achievement correlated significantly and positively correlation with socioeconomic status, knowledge value and occupational aspiration but negatively with power value. In the case of arts and science group student there is a significant correlation between academic achievement and socio-economic status but in the case of commerce group students there is no relation between these variables. Further **Trivedi, Vineeta (1988)** carried out a study of the relationship of parental attitude, socio-economic background and the feeling of security among the intermediate students and their academic background and found a significant correlation among parental attitude, socioeconomic status and academic achievement. Students belonging to various level of parental attitude and socio-economic status differed significantly with the parental acceptance group showing better achievement than parental concentration or avoidance groups. Further, students of upper SES showed better achievement than the students of lower SES group. There existed no significant relationship between feelings of security-insecurity, parental attitude and intelligence. **Andrew (1999)** stated that children from low socio-economic background have poorer mastery of English language (their second language) as it is used in schools than children from higher socioeconomic levels. **Edinyang, S. D. (2013)** found that the retention ability of higher SES students is significantly greater than that of medium SES students who in turn had significantly higher retention ability than low SES students. Based on these findings, recommendations were made. **Akhter and Pandey (2018)** found that male students of Secondary school perceived higher parental encouragement as compared to female students In Jammu and Kashmir.

2.1.3 SOCIO-ECONOMIC STATUS AND SELF-CONFIDENCE

Nagiach, 1987 stated that parenting style had a great influence on a personality development and disposition of the children. **Toddlers (1990)** found that when parents have high expectation, the child may develop low self-confidence. Further **Kumar and Kohli (2012)** conducted a study on the relationship between home environment and self-confidence among 200 students of secondary school students and found no significant relationship between protectiveness, punishment, conformity, reward, deprivation of privileges and permissiveness and self-confidence among adolescents. **Geetika (2017)** Found A Positive Relation In Parental Encouragement And Self-Confidence Among Adolescents In Punjab. **Filippin Antonio &Paccagnella Marco (2011)** found that there is a correlation between family background and self-confidence and that the learning process is slow: inherited beliefs about one's ability can survive a long string of signals. On the other side **Debrah, K., (2018) & Sang, C. C., (2015)**.revealed that there was no significant relationship between socio-economic status and self-esteem. Further **Dr. Meena (2015)** found that there is no significant difference in the self-confidence of male and female students who belong to high and low Socio-economic status and she also found that there is no significant difference in the self-confidence of male students belongs to high and Low Socio-economic status. In the study of **Weber (2001)** gender difference have been noted with boys Self-esteem being affected by the parental support more than the self-esteem of girls.

2.1.4. SOCIO-ECONOMIC STATUS AND MENTAL HEALTH

Melki, Beydoun, Khogali, Tamim, &Yunis, (2004) found that lower SES has been linked to domestic crowding which is a condition that has negative effect for adult and children, such as higher psychological stress and poor health outcomes. **(Newacheck, Hung, Park, Brindis, & Irwin, 2003)** also found that lower level of SES associate with higher rates of depression, anxiety, attempted suicide, cigarette dependence, illicit drug use, and episodic heavy drinking among adolescents. **Ikpaya (2004)** found that children who are economically depressed can develop certain psychological feelings which might lead to frustrating performance. Similar results were found by **Elgar FJ, Pfortner TK, Moor I, De Clercq B, Stevens GW, Currie C (2015)** which revealed that adolescents with a low SES are more affected by psychological and physical symptoms. **Reiss F. (2013)** found that Children and adolescents with low SES are two to three times more likely to develop mental health problems than their peers with high SES. Family income and education of parents have a great effect on the mental health problems of children and adolescents than parental unemployment or low occupation status, which refers to a low position in the occupational hierarchy. **Padilla-Moledo C, Ruiz JR, Castro-Pinero J. (2016)** found that parents with a university degree are more likely to have children with higher positive psychological health than children of parents with no university degree. Further **Glasscock DJ, Andersen JH, Labriola M, Rasmussen K, Hansen CD. (2013)** revealed that lower parental education and lower household income were associated with higher stress levels irrespective of adolescent's gender.

Further **Rozumah, Siti Nor, Rojanah and Abdullah al-hadi, 2013; Shak, 2011** found that family functionality can affect the development and wellbeing of the individual in term of emotionally, mentally and physically. **Bandhana and Sharma,**

Darshan, P. (2010) carried out a study on home environment, mental health and academic achievement among Hr. Secondary School students and found that there are significant differences in mental health among Secondary students with good and poor home environment. **Borkowsky, (2002),** clearly reveals the continued significance of parents in shaping the behavior and choice of adolescents as they face the challenges of growing up. **Manguvani E (1990)** found that the home environment is significant contributor to all components of mental health. Further **Rai and Yadav (1993)** revealed that Mental Health of low socio-economic status students is lower than that of the Students of higher socio-economic status. According to the family stress model of **V.C. Mcloyd et. al., (2009)** economic hardship negatively affects psychological adjustment of children indirectly through its impact on the parent's behavior towards the child". **Geeta S. Pastey G.S. and Aminbhavi V. A. (2006)** found out the effect of adolescent's emotional maturity on their stress and self-confidence. The findings revealed that the adolescents who have high emotional maturity also have significantly high stress and high self-confidence when compared to those with low emotional maturity. Adolescents with more number of siblings have shown significantly higher level of self-confidence than their counter parts. It is also found that father's educational level has significantly influenced the stress of their adolescent. Adolescent boys tend to have significantly higher stress than girls and girls tend to have significantly high self-confidence. **Conger et.al, (1994)** showed that financial strain increases parent's feeling of depression worsen marital relationship and increase family conflicts. These consequences negatively affects family relations. Negative family environment affect adolescents mental health negatively. The studies of **Elovainio et. al., 2012; Sichko et. al., (2015)** have been found that family context and internal resources are an important factors that are associated with adolescent's depression. **Bradley RH, Corwyn RF, (2002)** also revealed that low socio-economic status is associated with higher stress, worse parenting style and poor social environment. Low SES affect adolescent personality. In a study carried out by **Singh, Arun Kumar, Kumari Savita and Kumari Suprashna (2008)** on mental health behavior as function of SES and locality. 200 male and female college students participated in the study. 100 students were taken from rural areas and 100 students were taken from urban area colleges of Patna District. The mental health battery and SES scale were administered on them. The analyses was done with the help of t-test. The results revealed that lower SES had a negative impact upon sound development of mental health behavior. However, urban rural region was not found to be a significant determiner of mental health behavior. On the other side a study was carried out by **Srividhya, V.; and Khadi, Pushpa, B (2007)** on mental health and adjustment problems of students from Navodhaya, central and state schools and found that Age, type of family, ordinal position, sibling status and constellation, parent's education and occupation and income of family did not affect mental health and adjustment problems. Transition from school to college in case of state schools had no influence. Mental health was significantly correlated to adjustment problems which indicate that if the adjustment problems is high than the mental health will be low. While **Anand, S.P. (1989)** indicated that adolescents' mental health , academic achievement and the educational and occupational status of parents were positively correlated.

Many researchers like **DeCarlo Santiago, Wadsworth, & Stump, 2011; Russell, Ford, Williams & Russell, 2016; Spencer, Kohn & Woods, 2002,** found that Low level of SES are associate with High level of emotional and behavioral difficulties, such as social problems, delinquent behavior symptoms and attention deficit among adolescents. **Abdur Rahman, ArunavoBairagi, BiplobKumaDey (2014)** showed that gender and SES have significant effect on adolescent anger, male express more anger than female with low SES than middle and high SES. **Molnar, Cerda, Roberts, & Buka (2008)** also found that Lower level of SES are associated with higher level of aggression. **Dev et al (2015)** conducted a study on "role of the home environment, parental care, and parent's personality on adolescent mental health with a focus on adjustment, anxiety, self-concept, and self-confidence. Parental traits were found to negatively influence mental health, anxiety, adjustment, self-concept, and Self-confidence.

2.1.5. SOCIO-ECONOMIC STATUS AND PERSONAL VALUES

Nagrajan Pavithra, Ahuja Abha and Singh Ritu (2020), found that family income plays a crucial role in the personal values of adolescents. **Robert REL, Bengtson VL. (1999),** also stated that families are an important factor for the development of children's values. Further **Blais (2010)** found that personal values develops through being affected by family, culture, society, environment, religious belief and ethnicity. But on the other hand **Benish- Weisman et. al., (2017)** found that in adolescence period, adolescents are more influenced by their peers then by parents.

S.M. Shahidul , A.H.M. Zehadul Karim and S.M.A. Suffiun (2016) found that students from lower class family background have much more religious value rather than the students from higher class family background. Conversely, students from higher class family background have much more democratic and power values rather than the the students from lower class background. Furthermore, though some values vary in class backgrounds of students but there is no significant difference in them. Further **Magre Sunita (2011)** revealed that there was a significance difference in the religious, democratic, economic, knowledge, hedonistic, family prestige and health values of high socio-economic status and low socioeconomic status of the students of high socio-economic status found to be higher on religious values whereas students of low socio-economic status were found to be higher on democratic, economic, knowledge, hedonistic, power, family prestige. On the other hand **Atul Madaan and J. Senthil Kumaran (2015)** revealed that there is no significant difference in personal values and coping among the adolescents of different type of families. There is a significant correlation between personal values and coping of the respondents. The findings of the study further shows that there is a significant correlation between coping strategies and moral values of adolescents which involved in pre-marital sex.

According to **Devi, B. (2000)**, Degradation of values among adolescents is caused by the responsibility of family. **Mittal, A. (2016)**, found that socio-economic status had a significant effect on the religious, social, family prestige and health values of the students. **Verma, D. (1996)**, in his study on value pattern of 400 college students of Rohilkhand region with special reference to sense of responsibility, reflected that social values were higher among arts students and theoretical values among science and commerce students. The study further reported that the socio-economic status did not affect the values of college students and the streams of study (arts, science and commerce) did not differ significantly in their sense of responsibility.

2.2 STUDIES ON SELF-CONFIDENCE

Various studies have been conducted on the self-confidence of adolescents with different variables. An effort has been made by the researcher by the study adolescent's self-confidence under the following sub-headings.

4. Locality, school and gender difference among adolescents self-confidence.
5. Self-confidence and academic achievement. /

6. Self-confidence and mental health

2.2.1 LOCALITY, SCHOOL AND GENDER DIFFERENCE AMONG ADOLESCENTS SELF-CONFIDENCE.

Wankhade and Rokade (2011) conducted a comparative study on self-confidence of rural and urban students of Amrawati city which were studying in 8th standard of various schools of Amravati. They found that there were no difference in self-confidence of rural and urban, boys and girls but the rural boys had more self-confidence rather than the rural girls and the self-confidence of both sexes of urban areas were almost same. **Fareen Fatma (2015)** found significant difference between urban and rural adolescents in relation to their self-confidence and also found a significant difference between the academic achievement of urban and rural adolescents. It also found positive correlation between self-confidence and academic achievement of adolescents. Similar result was found by **S.M. Makvana., (2012)** which revealed that urban male, students of higher Secondary are more developed with respect to self-confidence compared to rural female secondary school students. Further **Purwar (2002)** investigated the self-confidence, intelligence & level of aspirations among urban and rural schedule caste boys and girls. The results revealed that self-confidence was positively and significantly correlated.

Baghla (2004): Conducted a study on the effect of socio emotional climate of school on self-confidence of students. From her studies she concluded that- male and female students do not differ in their self-confidence and type of sex and school interacted significantly on the self-confidence of students. **Thakur (2008):** Reported that the students of public school have more self-confidence followed by the students of central and govt. schools. Although type of sex does not influence the self-confidence of the students, whereas type of school influences. Further **Dr. Anshu Narad , Amit Kumar Singh (2020),** revealed that the girls from Private Schools had more Self-Confidence as compared to girls from government school. They further found that Government And Private Schools' girl received similar encouragement from their parents and there is a significant and positive relation exists between Self-Confidence And parental encouragement of senior secondary school girls. **Verma, R.K. and KumariSaroj (2016)** found no significant difference in the self-confidence of male and female elementary school students. It was also found that there exists a significant difference in the academic achievement of elementary school students with high and low self-confidence. **Vyas and Gunthey (2017)** also reported no significant difference in self-confidence in relation to gender. Further **Ghaonta (2015)** revealed that School students did not differ in self-confidence w.r.t. their gender and area. Students differed significantly in self-confidence w.r.t. their stream. Gender x stream had combined effect on self-confidence of school students at 0.05 level of significance. Gender x stream x area had no combined effect on self-confidence of school students even at 0.05 level of significance. **Prajapati, K. (2019)** also found that there is no significant difference between the self-confidence of college students with relation to their Gender and stream.

On the other side **Singh & Kaur (2008)** observed that gender has a significant effect on self-confidence. **Malhotra & Malhotra (2016)** examined the main and interactional effect of students and showed that self-confidence was found to be associated with gender, locality and type of school. Further **DuBois, Burk, Braston, Swenson, Tevandale and Hardesty (2002)** found that race, gender and environment plays an important role in the course of development of adolescent's self-confidence. Similar result was found by **Dr. Jyoti Prasad (2015)**, which indicated that there were no significant differences in the Self Concept of boys and girls and urban and rural adolescents but found a significant gender differences in Self Confidence score. The girls had significantly high Self Confidence rather than the boys. **Lal Krishan (2014)**, found that there were a significant difference between male and female adolescents on emotional maturity. Female adolescents are higher on self-confidence in comparison to male adolescents. **Renu Tomer R. and Agrawal A. (2014)** found that parental deprivation and gender significantly affect the self-confidence of adolescents after exploring the effect of parental deprivation on self-confidence of adolescents. The result reveals that **Ziegler *et al.* (2000)** reported that girls expressed significantly low self-confidence as compared to boys. **Kou (2003):** Found that the self-confidence was negatively correlated with cognitive state anxiety, somatic state anxiety and trait anxiety. Male weight lifters had high self-confidence than female weight lifters. The international athlete's self-confidence was higher than local athlete's self-confidence.

2.2.2. SELF-CONFIDENCE AND ACADEMIC ACHIEVEMENT

Norman and Hyland (2003), found that most of the problems in the educational system is due to lack of self-confidence in students that lead a number of students having lack of enough participation and unsatisfactory progress. **Fareen Fatma (2015)**

found that there was a positive correlation between self-confidence and academic achievement of adolescents. **Rathee & Sheetal (2017)** also found A Positive correlation in Self-Confidence and Academic Achievement of Secondary School Students. Similarly **Singh. Y.G., (2010),** revealed that the significant co-relationship between self- confidence & academic achievement. Further **Lal. K. (2014)** found that there is significant relationship between self-confidence and academic achievement of male and female adolescents. **Srimadevi and Saraladevi (2016)** identified that decision making and self-confidence has an impact on problem solving ability among mathematics achievers. **Nowicki ad Duke (1992)** found that low levels of empathy, handling stress, self-confidence, self-acceptance, group dynamics and control on emotions were associated with poor achievement. Further **Verma, R.K. and Kumari Saroj (2016)** findings of the study revealed that significant relationship exists between self-confidence and academic achievement of elementary school students. **Dr. Malik & Yougesh (2014),** also revealed that there is a significant difference among academic achievement of 11th class students with high and low self-confidence.

On the other hand Maikhuri**, R. and Panole, S.K. (1977)** revealed that there is no significant correlation between academic achievement and self-confidence. However significant differences were observed in the academic achievement of the high and low self-confidence group. Further **Saini (2016)** explored the self-confidence and academic achievement of students and found no significant interactional effect with respect to gender and type of family. **Tandon, Uma (1994)** carried out a comparative study of self-concept among high and normal IQ adolescents in relation to creativity, SES and academic achievement and found that Self-concept was significantly related to intelligence and creativity. Self-concept was found to be to be significantly related with academic achievement only under uncontrolled conditions but uncorrelated under controlled conditions. Self-concept was not related with SES. Creatively was found to be significantly correlated with intelligence and academic achievement. The effect of sex was found to be highly significant between creativity and intelligence and creativity and academic achievement and boys were found to be more intensely related than girls. **Still, Pulford & Sohal (2006)** explore self-confidence of students on academic abilities by measuring individual's learning profile. Their findings revealed that students' carefulness, honesty, and the attitude of expecting everything to be perfect are an important factors which influence students' academic confidence and also affected students' confidence.

2.2.3 SELF-CONFIDENCE AND MENTAL HEALTH

Due to low self-confidence many psychological barriers such as feelings of insecurity, fearfulness, anxiety and feeling yourself apart from the society are an important barriers that arise during the class which can negatively affects the performance of students. They can consequently be leading an individual being distracted from the learning process. According to personal experiences of different researchers, it is found that most of students of Kandahar University having poor participation in classes. **Rubio (2007)** found that participation is closely related to self-confidence, this is the major concern that students' poor performance maybe due to the lack of self-confidence which can consequently affect their vulnerability in learning process. **(Rosenberg M. et.al., 1995)** found that depression and anxiety are associated with self-esteem. Similarly **Mann et. al., (2004)** stated that there is a role of self-esteem in the development of mental disorders and social problems such as depression, anxiety and violence. So a relationship has also been found between self-esteem and anxiety level many researchers **Erol and Orth, 2011; Riaz and Sarwat, 2013; Lee and Hankin, 2009,** found that an increase in self-esteem result in a decline of internal and reactive anxiety and vice versa.

Neelima, M. (2013). Found a positive correlation between self-confidence and mental health. **Selvaraj and Gnanadevan (2014)** conducted a study on self-confidence and stress among higher secondary students of Cuddalore District of Tamil Nadu This study reveals that there is a significant and negative correlation between self-confidence and different dimensions of stress such as, academic stress, interpersonal stress, intrapersonal stress, environmental stress and total stress. Further **Tikkoo, Sangeeta (2006)** studied introversion and mental health among school students and revealed that where extroversion tendency enhances mental health, introversion tendency deteriorates it. **Patterson and Capaldi, 1992,** found that low self-esteem can increase one's risk of developing an eating disorder, depression, and/or anxiety. The clinical literature suggests that low self-esteem is related to depressed moods. A significant and negative relationship is found between self-esteem and depression by many studies. **(Beck *et al.*, 1990; Patton, 1991). Beck *et al.*, (2001)** found that self-esteem to be inversely correlated with anxiety and other signs of psychological and physical distress. Likewise, **Solomon *et al.*, (2000)** revealed that bolstering self-esteem in adults reduces anxiety.

Further Carvajal *et al.*, (1998), found that adolescents having more positive self-concepts are less likely to use alcohol or drugs. **Fardouly, Jasmine; Vartanian, Lenny R. (June 2016)** found that Both adolescent boys and girls are impacted by the objectifying nature of social media, however young girls are more likely to body surveil due to society's tendency to overvalue and objectify women. **Zimmerman, (2000)** found that self-esteem has significant variance in both mental well-being and happiness. **Goel M. and Aggarwal P (2012)** reported self Confidence is one of the personality trait which is a composite of a person's thoughts and feelings, strivings and hopes, fears and fantasies, his view of what he is, what he has been, what he might become, and his attitudes pertaining to his worth. They further described self Confidence as the ability of an individual to tackle situations successfully without leaning on others to have a positive self-evaluation. They also reported that a self-confident person perceives himself to be socially competent. He is emotionally mature, intellectually and adequately successful. He is also satisfied, optimistic, independent, decisive, self-reliant, self-assured, forward moving, fairly assertive and having leadership qualities.

2.3 STUDIES ON MENTAL HEALTH

Adolescence is the developmental stage of life of an individual. It is also recognized as a period of crucial development due to many stresses and strains. Now-a-day, adolescents are facing many difficulties in life that are giving rise to many psychosomatic problems such as anxiety, tension, frustration and depression. The environmental factors indicates that socio-economic status, self-confidence, home environment, school environment etc. all play significant role in the mental health development of adolescents.

Many studies have been conducted on the mental health of adolescents with different variables. It was not possible for the researcher to survey all of the available literature. But an effort has been made by the researcher to study adolescent's mental health under the following sub-headings.

5. Locality, school and gender difference among adolescents mental health
6. Mental health and academic achievement
7. Emotional maturity and emotional stability
8. Adjustment level

2.3.1 LOCALITY, SCHOOL AND GENDER DIFFERENCE AMONG ADOLESCENTS MENTAL HEALTH

Mittal A. (2008) found no significant difference in mental health of secondary level students of rural as well as urban localities. **Singh, Arun kumar, Kumari Savita and Kumari Suprashna (2008)** also found that urban rural reason was not a significant determiner of mental health behavior. Further **Doering Lynn V.; Eastwood, Jo-Ann (2011)** found that Regardless of one's age and country of origin, women are more likely to have depression than men. **Srividhya, V.; and Khadi, Pushpa, B (2007)** carried out a study on mental health and adjustment problems of students of Navodhaya, central and state schools and found that there were no difference in the mental health status of Boys and girls. Significantly, higher percentage of girls of central school and boys of Navodhadya had positive mental health. **Singh, B., Kumar, A. & Moral, A. (2015)** carried out a study in which they compared the mental health of male and female students. For testing the hypotheses, a sample of 346 students of age group of 16 to 23 years, was used to collect the data. Results showed that there is no significant difference between the mental health scores of male and female students. There was also no correlation between gender and mental health. Similar result was found by **Dr. Bhagat Singh 2016** which revealed no significant difference among mental health of male and female students. On the other hand **Quadri & Akolkar (2011)** found that there was significant difference between male and female college going students. Significance difference was not found between rural and urban colleg'e going students. There was no interaction effect of area of residence and gender on mental health in college going students. Similarly **Bandhana and Sharma, (2010)** carried out a study on home environment, mental health and academic achievement among Hr. secondary school students. There are significant sex differences in mental health among secondary school Students. Girls are more mentally healthy in comparison to boys.

Santosh, L. et al., (2009) show that men have better mental health than women. Similar result was found by **Singh, S., (2015),** Which revealed that male group was mentally healthy than female group. Further **Dooner, Nina; Lowry, Christopher (May 2014)** found that Women are two to three times more likely to be diagnosed with General Anxiety Disorder (GAD) than men and have higher self-reported anxiety scores. **World Health Organization** found that Gender is correlated with certain mental disorders, such as depression, anxiety and somatic complaints. For example, women are more likely to have major depression, while men are more likely to have substance abuse and antisocial personality disorder. **Legy, 2018** also found that women are more likely to be diagnostic with anxiety disorders as compared to man. Similarly **Zareena et. al, (1988)** conducted a study on a sample of 725 adolescents and concluded that more no of females were in high anxiety group than males. **Manjuvani E. (1990)** carried out a study on influence of home and school environment on the mental health status of children. The school environment contributed to liabilities and the mental health index. **Chaing (1995)** proposed that school is one of the main source of stress among adolescents such stress come from too much homework,, preparation for test, lack of interest in particular subject and teacher punishment. **Sarita, Rajni, and Pushpanjali (2015)** found that there is significant difference in mental health of boys as well as girls of government and private senior secondary schools. They further found that there is no significant difference in mental health of boys and girls of government senior secondary schools as well as private senior secondary schools. **Bala Subramaniam (1994)** reported that the male students studying in private schools have higher level of achievement anxiety than female students. On the other side **Reddy S., Prasad K. and Md. Hamza Ameer (2015)** revealed that students from government and private schools do not have any significant difference in their self-esteem and stress. Students from both school had low level of stress and normal level of self-esteem.

Singh, B., Kumar, A. & Moral, A. (2014) showed that there was a significant difference between the mental health of art, science and commerce faculty students. **Kunal Kishor Jha, et.al. (2017)** showed that of the 1412 respondents surveyed, 49.2 percent of them were suffering from moderate depression and 7.7 percent of them were suffering from severe depression. The study also found that there is a significant difference in depression with regard to girls and boys. It shows that girls had higher prevalence of mental health problems compared to boys.

2.3.2 MENTAL HEALTH AND ACADEMIC ACHIEVEMNT

Bandhana and Sharma, (2010) carried out a study on home environment, mental health and academic achievement among Hr. secondary school students and found that there were insignificant differences in mental health of high and low academic achievement students of secondary school. **Mittal, A. (2008)** carried out a study on academic achievement of secondary level students in relation to mental health and locality and found that the secondary level Students of different localities were different in their academic achievement. Secondary level students of urban areas have good academic achievement as compared to secondary level students of rural areas. The difference between mental health of secondary level students of different localities is significant. He further found that there is no significant difference in mental health of secondary level students of rural as well as urban areas. The relationship between academic achievement and mental health of students of secondary level of urban locality is highly significant. There is a high significant relationship between academic achievement and mental health of secondary level students of rural locality but there is no significant difference between academic achievement and mental health of secondary level students of different localities. Moreover, depression is associated with negative results, including academic difficulties interpersonal dysfunction as well as health problems **(Berndt et. al., 2000; Zlotnick et. al., 2000). Singh and Singh (1986),** conducted that anxiety and intelligence were negatively correlated.

Singh, S., (2015). Revealed that mental health was positively related with academic achievement. The group which had high academic achievement was mentally healthy than low achiever group. **Agnafors, S. et al. (2020)** found that mental health problems in early childhood and adolescence increase the risk for poor academic performance. Many researchers **Robbins et al., 2004; Storrie et al., 2010,** have reported that emotional problems had a negative effect on study progress and on the dropout rate from higher education. **Keyes et al., (2012)** found that anxiety and depression are harmful for academic and social participation in everyday student life. **Rice et al., (2006) and Stallmann, (2008)** further revealed that depression and anxiety often affect memory and concentration, which makes it more difficult to acquire new knowledge and cope with examination situations. **RadhikaKapur (2020)** reported that when anxiety takes place in a major form, it has deter mental effects upon health and well-being of the individuals.

2.3.3 EMOTIONAL MATURITY AND EMOTIONAL STABILITY

According to **Hay & Ashman, 2003,** an emotional stability may be indicated as calmness of mind and freedom from anxiety and depression. **Natesan and Devi (1987),** conducted a comparative study of the personality of high and low academic achievers among sixty girls of XIth standard it was found that high and low achievers differed significantly in the trades i.e. emotional stability, boldness and self-assurance. **Bindo, (2016)** found that the students in rolled the government and the private schools have similar emotional stability label. On the other side **Dr. Chitra Sharma (2017)** found that there is significant difference in emotional stability of boys and girls of government school and private schools. Government school students are more emotionally stable that the private school students. The girls from private school are more emotionally stable as compared to boys from private school. Government school boys is more emotionally stable than the govt. school girls. Government school boys are more emotionally stable than the private school boys. Government school girls are emotionally stable than the private school girls. Further **Mahajan and Sharma (2008)** revealed that girls were found more emotionally unstable then boys, whereas anxiety and mental tension was found more in boys. **Singh (1989)** explored sex linked traits of intelligent youth in a sample of four hundred and eighty youths. Results showed that high intelligent males scored significantly high on emotional stability, conscientiousness, tender mindedness and suspiciousness while female averaged as shrewd. Less intelligent males were emotionally unstable, assertive, experimentally, imaginative, and tensed, the females being outgoing and apprehensive.

Study conducted by **Kaur (2001)** found that there is a significant relationship between emotional maturity and parental encouragement. Boys and girls did not differ significantly in their emotional maturity. Similar result was found by **Anju, (2000)** which revealed that emotional maturity level of the senior secondary school students (boys and girls) of the Chandigarh is almost same. Further **Ritu Singh (2013)** revealed that girls scored significantly higher on the social adequacy component of social maturity whereas boys scored significantly higher on the social adjustment component of emotional maturity. **Manjeet Kaur (2013)** supported that there is significant difference in various areas of emotional maturity of govt. and private school students; no significant difference in the emotional maturity level of boys and girls of senior secondary schools of Chandigarh found. **Mahendra, Rajni and Ravindra Kumar (2018)** also found that the student of government school have high emotional majority than that of private school students. There is no significant difference between the emotional maturity of government girls and private school girls. The emotional maturity of government school boys are higher than that of private school boys. **Singh, Thukral (2011)** found that there is no significant relationship between emotional maturity and academic achievement. While a significant relationship between emotional maturity and academic achievement was found in case of boys but no significant relationship was found between the two variables in a case of girls. **Dharamvir et al. (2011)** a study by the data obtained was analysed statistically and the study reveals that there is no significant difference in anxiety & emotional maturity among adolescents' girls and boys studying from co-educational and educational schools.

Gosh (2003) conducted a study on academic achievement, self-conception and emotional maturity of male and female adolescents and found that there is no significant difference between the emotional maturity level of male and female adolescents. **Pavlenko, Chernyi and Goubkina, (2009)** found that attributes of emotional maturity, self-confidence, and stability in their plans and affections are found in the one who is emotional stable. **Ranjit.L and Natarajan.P. (2013)** revealed that a moderate level of emotional autonomy was found among the respondents. The study also concludes that demographic variables like age, gender, type of family, family size and mothers" education do influence the level of emotional autonomy of the respondent.

2.3.4 AJDUSTMENT LEVEL

According to A**.K. Menninger** mental health is an adjustment of human being to the world and to each other with a maximum of effectiveness and happiness. **Mudasir, 2013,** defined that mental health is a condition and a level of function which is socially acceptable and personally satisfied. **Srividhya and Puspha (2007)** carried out studies on mental health and adjustment problems of students of Navodaya, Central and state schools and found that mental health was significantly correlated to adjustments problems indicating higher the problems, lower the mental health. **Bhatia (1992)** investigated the significant effect of anxiety and adjustment level of male and female degree college students in age range of 18-22 years. He concluded that anxiety has a significant impact on the level of adjustment in all areas i.e. home, emotional, educational and social. **Mehta et. al. 2005** found that sex had significant effect upon social and emotional adjustment of adolescents. Girls were better adjusted then boys. Similar results were obtained by **Godiyal and Padiyar (2008),** which showed that boys and girls differed significantly in their adjustment. Girls were very superior to boys in their educati onal and emotional adjustment, whereas both boys and girls were poorly adjusted to their social lives. Further **Veena and Khadi (2004)** also revealed that girls were well adjusted both emotionally and at home. Boys were socially and educationally well adjusted. On the other side **Bhatt (2007)** revealed that the boy and girl students have same level of total adjustment.

Hussain et al (2008) indicates that magnitude of academic stress was significantly higher among the private school students whereas Government school students were significantly better in terms of their level of adjustment. **Babu (2004)** found significant difference between the rural students and urban students in respect to their adjustment. **Rout, Manisa and Mantry, Sudhir Kumar (2011)** carried out a study of academic achievement of secondary school children in relation to their self-confidence and adjustment and found that there is no significant difference between adjustment of students having high Academic achievement, average academic achievement and low academic achievement. The study also found that there was significant difference between adjustment of male and female students at secondary level.

2.4 STUDIES ON PERSONAL VALUES

Personal values of an individual are related to their choice. He makes decision and choose behaviour, friends, jobs etc. on the basis of his personal values. There is a lot of confusion in the minds of adolescents about what to believe, how to believe, what to follow and what type of life style to copy. The paradox is that while parents offer one set of values and society proposes another set of moralization. Personal values affects various aspects of an individual's life. Many studies have been conducted on personal values which are studied by the researcher under the following sub-headings.

4. Effect of personal values
5. Academic achievement and personal values
6. Locality, gender difference and type of school among adolescents personal values

2.4.1 EFFECT OF PERSONAL VALUES

According to **Theodorson and Achilles, 1969,** personal values or individual values are those values to which an individual is committed and which affects his behavior. Personal values are implicitly related to individual choice. We make decisions and choose behaviors, friends, jobs and hobbies according to our personal values **(Verma and Panwar)**. **Kasai, K., Fukuda M., (2017)** stated that personal values is a broad goal, varying in importance, underlying, guiding attitudes and behavior. Adolescence is a developmental stage during which differentiation of personal values progress **(Daniel et., 2012)**. **Converse (1965)** stated that values can be considered as the ultimate development of those many process of selection and generalized that produce long range consistency and organization in individuals. **Boyce et. al., (2013)** said that Values influence the person's behavior and attitude and gives suitable guidelines in all situations. When particular values are strong and silent to individuals, they are generally motivated to behave in ways that one consistent with their goals.

The relationship between personality traits and personal values was also studied by **Olver (2003),** the study indicated that personal values were affected in predicted pattern by Openness/intellect, Agreeableness and Conscientiousness as well as more moderately by extraversion. **Pradhan, G. C. (1997)** conducted a study to explore the relationship between moral values with 10 personal values of 561 boy and girl school students of Puri district (Orissa). The results of Pearson's correlation revealed that moral judgement was positively correlated with religious, social, knowledge and health values, and was negatively correlated with personal and family-prestige values. **Rosenbaum et. al. (2014)** found that women cheat less than men.

2.4.2 ACADEMIC ACHIEVEMENT AND PERSONAL VALUES

Gupta (1992) designed his study to assess the academic satisfaction of graduate students as related to their personality needs and personal values and found that academic satisfaction was significantly related to their personality needs and personal values. **Susan and Ansupama (1998),** found that high academic achievers had higher values than the low achievers. **Khatun and Halder (2019)** found a positive correlation between personal values and academic achievement of higher secondary students. Further **Matthews (2004)** showed that values were related to different approaches to learning. **Bala (2014)** explored that high and low achievers were similar of religious value.**Jafri, Bilkis Sultana (1992)** in her comparative study of Values and Aspirations of undergraduate women students between two colleges, found that the students of Arts Stream of Tika Ram College were significantly higher in values as compared to the students of Women's college, while the aspirations of students of Women's College was higher as compared to the students Tika Ram College. The study also revealed the existence of significant difference in the aspiration and values between arts and science students, between high and low educated parental groups as well as between high and low parental income groups.

2.4.3 LOCALITY, GENDER DIFFERENCE AND TYPE OF SCHOOL AMONG ADOLESCENTS PERSONAL VALUES

Benjamin, B. Maxwell (2011) conducted a study to find out the prevalence of moral judgement among higher secondary school students of Chennai city with respect to classification of different school climate and home environment. The findings revealed that the school students in high school climate had higher moral, personal, social, aesthetic, humanitarian and religious values than the students in moderate and low school climate. On the other hand, in all these values the scores among the students of moderate and low school climates were similar. Contrary to this, the academic value was found similar among school students irrespective of the level of school climate. With regard to the influence of home environment, the study showed that in moral, personal, academic, social and aesthetic values students were similar irrespective of the level of home environment (high, moderate and low), whereas in humanitarian and religious values the students of low home environment were significantly higher than the students of high and moderate home environment.

Vasuki (2003), showed that there is a significant effect of gender, locality, type and system of school on the values of the students. **Kaur (1998)** found that the adolescents' from joint families were found higher score on moral value in comparison to adolescents from nuclear families and also found that girls from joint families had higher moral values in comparison to adolescent boys from joint families. Further **Shah, H. M. (1992)** made an investigation into the values of higher secondary school students of Saurashtra. In this study Shah showed that sex, residential area, stream of the study had significant relationship with the values of students studying in class XI and XII. The study further revealed that stream or branch of study was significantly related to social value. **Verma, Rajalakshmi and Swain, (1993)** in their study of the main effect of sex and rural/urban inhabitation on the values of adolescent students found that male adolescents had high on truth, non-violence and love value than female adolescents but there were no significant difference between male and female adolescents with respect to right conduct value and peace value. Again, on the variable of inhabitation all the F-ratios were found highly significant.

Christensen (1992) reported significant sex differences in values as measured by the Rokeach value survey. He found that males ranked the values of loyalty and ambition higher than the females. **Ismail, H. (2015)** showed that females plays a higher weight on personal values such as "ethics" and "citizenship", while males put a stronger emphasis on "masculinity". Further **Dr. Nasir Ali1 and Dr. Fakhruddin Ali Ahmad (2018)** found that there is no significant difference on religious value, knowledge value, hedonistic value, power value, family prestige value and health value of girls and boys whereas two groups differed significantly on Social Value, democratic value, aesthetic value and economic value. Adolescent boys showed significantly more attitude towards social value as compared to adolescent girls. On the other hand, adolescent girls showed significantly more attitudes towards democratic value, aesthetic value and economic value as compared to adolescent boys. On the other side **Manivannan (2003),** revealed that gender did not have an impact on the attitudes of students towards values. **Gupta (2002)** found that they there were significant difference in the values of students studying in government and private schools. Further **N. Rani (2009)** stated that urban girls have high moral values than rural girls. Government school students have high moral values than private school students. Similar result was obtained by **Malti (2006)** which revealed that the students of UP board schools have been found to have higher social and knowledge values than the students of CBSE board schools. **Dr. Mamta Taneja (2017)** also found a significant difference between the moral values of government and private school students. The moral values of government school students is higher than the private school students. The result also revealed that the female students have high moral values than male students of secondary school.

Natasha (2013) reported that urban and rural adolescents both gave first importance to social values because both are resourceful and can translate virtues like love, sympathy and kindness into their behaviour. They gave second preference to political values. **Nidhi and Jyoti (2011)** revealed that the college students showed very high attitude for economic values, power values, aesthetic values and hedonistic values whearse average attitude was noticed towards religious, and family prestige values, lower were seen for democratic, knowledge and health values and lowest for social value. **Bhatia (2013)** conducted a study on personal values of secondary school students. Personal values of a person develop by experience and interaction with others. It directs and guides client's choices later in life. It is interesting to find that the secondary schools students have high religious, democratic, economic, power and family prestige value whereas the students have low social, knowledge, hedonistic and health value.

2.5 HYPOTHESIS OF THE STUDY

From the above cited reviews of related literature it is very clear that in respect of gender, locality and type of school, adolescent's socio-economic status relationship with self-confidence, mental health and personal values were neither consistent nor conclusive. In case of relationship between self-confidence and mental health; self-confidence and personal values; personal values and mental health, a very few studies were available. In face not even a single study was found showing actual relationship between personal values and self-confidence and between personal values and mental health. Therefore, no general conclusion can be drawn. However, all these variables were identified as the significant predictors of adolescent's all-round development. Thus, this study departs from the previous researches.

Therefore, to arrive at meaningful conclusions and to achieve the objectives of the study, the researcher has tried to use as much a rigorous design as possible. As the study is exploratory in nature, therefore following null hypothesis were formulated.

1. There exists no significance differences between different dimensions of socio-economic status and self-confidence of adolescents.
2. There exists no significant differences of different dimensions of socio-economic status on mental health of adolescents.
3. There exists no significant differences of different dimensions of socio-economic status on personal values of adolescents.
4. There exists is no significant relationship between self-confidence and mental health of adolescents.
5. There exists is no significant relationship between self-confidence and personal values of adolescents.
6. There exists is no significant relationship between mental health and personal values of adolescent.
7. Locality does not affect self-confidence, mental health and personal values of adolescents.
8. No significant differences are obtained between self-confidence, mental health and personal values of adolescent when comparison is made on the basis of gender.
9. Types of school has null effect on self-confidence, mental health and personal values of adolescents.

CHAPTER-III
DESIGN OF THE STUDY

3.1 RESEARCH QUESTIONS

The present study proceed with the assumption that the socio-economic status of the adolescents of both the genders (girl and boy) from different localities (rural and urban) and from different types of school (Government and Non-Government) may be related to their self-confidence, personal values and mental health. In this context, the basic questions studied in the present study are:

1. Does the socio-economic statue of family affect the self-confidence, personal values and mental health of the adolescents?
2. Does the adolescent's gender, locality and type of school affect their self-confidence, personal values and mental health?
3. Is there any relationship between self-confidence, mental health and personal values of adolescents?

6.2 METHOD OF THE STUDY

After the researcher has selected the problem for study it is necessary to determine what method for collections of data is more suitable in solving the problem or in verifying hypothesis formulated. So for this study **"The Normative Survey Method"** was selected.

The normative survey method investigates, describes and interprets what exists at present. It involves events that have already taken place and may be related to the present condition.

3.3 POPULATION

Dehradun District of Uttarakhand State is divided into 6 blocks:-

1. Chakrata
2. Kalsi
3. Vikasnagar
4. Sahaspur
5. Raipur
6. Doiwala

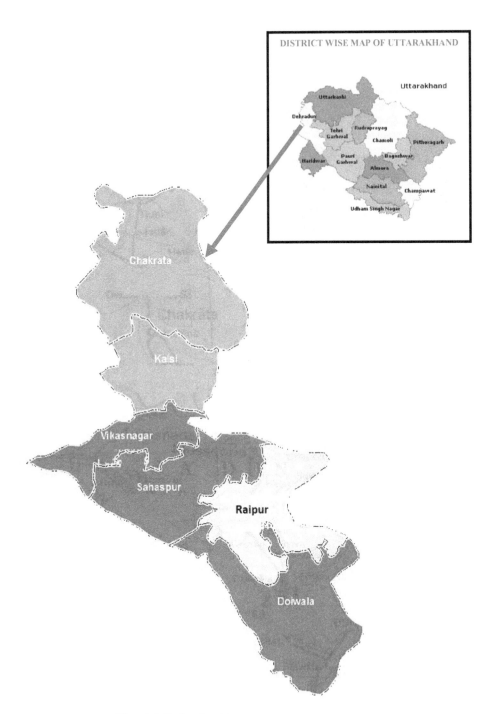

Fig:- 3.1: Dehradun District Block wise: Area of Study

All the adolescents studying in class XI and XII in the intermediate colleges of Dehradun District have been taken as the population for this study. There are a total number of 364 intermediate colleges in Dehradun District having a total of 54,242 adolescents studying in class XI and XII. The Gender wise, locality wise and school wise distribution of these inter colleges and adolescents are shown in Table 3.1 & 3.2 respectively.

The population consisted of all senior secondary school students who are studying in government and non-government schools of Dehradun district of Uttarakhand.

TABLE- 3.1

Gender wise, locality wise and school wise distribution of inter colleges among different block of Dehradun District.

Dehradun District	Number of Inter Colleges						
	Gender Wise			Locality Wise		School Wise	
Blocks	Boys School	Girls School	Co-Educated School	Rural	Urban	Govt. School	Non-Government School
Chakrata	-	01	17	18	-	17	1
Kalsi	-	02	13	15	-	14	1
Vikasnagar	-	1	37	29	9	18	20
Sahaspur	3	9	70	50	32	33	49
Raipur	8	17	119	39	105	61	83
Doiwala	6	4	57	50	17	32	35
Total	17	34	313	201	163	175	189

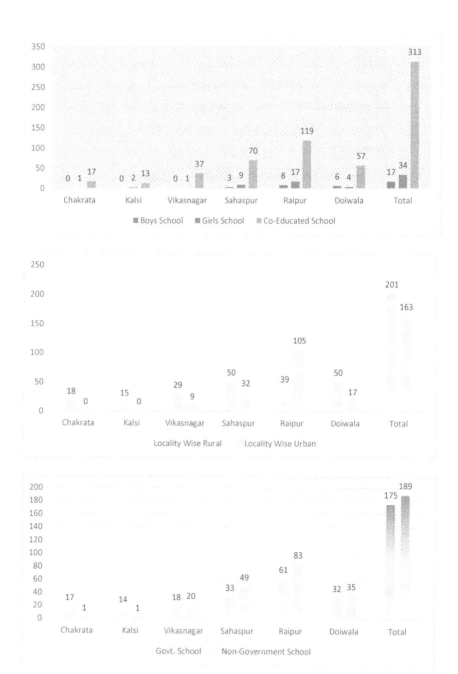

FIG: 3.2

Gender wise, Locality Wise and School Wise Distribution of Intermediate Colleges in Different Development Blocks of Dehradun District.

TABLE- 3.2

Gender wise, Locality Wise and School Wise Distribution of adolescents studying in XI and XII classes of Inter College among Different Developmental Blocks of Dehradun District.

Dehradun District	Number of Adolescents					
	Gender Wise		Locality Wise		School Wise	
Development Blocks	Boys	Girls	Rural	Urban	Govt. School	Non- Govt. School
Chakrata	666	850	1566	-	1475	91
Kalsi	534	851	1435	-	1316	119
Vikasnagar	3197	3247	5242	1176	3581	2837
Sahaspur	5317	4720	6498	3513	4284	5727
Raipur	12889	10646	3421	20088	7793	15716
Doiwala	6155	5170	7870	3433	5504	5799
Total	28758	25484	26032	28210	23953	30289

Source: From the records available at office of Zila Siksha Adhikari, MayurVihar Dehradun.

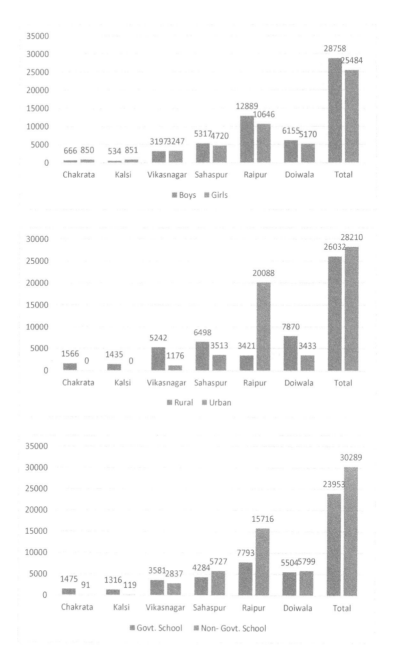

Fig:- 3.3

Gender wise, Locality Wise and School Wise Distribution of adolescents studying in XI and XII classes of Inter College among Different Developmental Blocks of Dehradun District.

3.4 SAMPLE AND SAMPLING TECHNIQUE

Keeping in view the objectives of this study as well as the size of the population, a stratified – random- sampling techniques was adopted to draw an adequate and representative sample for this study. In the first phase, out of six developmental blocks only four were selected on the basis of randomization (Lottery method) i.e., Vikasnagar, Sahaspur, Raipur and Doiwala. At the second phase, 88 Inter-College were chosen randomly from the total population 331 inter-colleges of Vikasnagar, Sahaspur, Raipur and Doiwala Blocks.

TABLE- 3.3

Gender wise, locality wise and School Wise of distribution of Inter colleges selected from the 4 Randomly Chosen Blocks of Dehradun District.

Dehradun District Blocks	Number of Inter Colleges							
	Gender Wise			Locality Wise		School Wise	
	Boys School	Girls School	Co-Educated School	Rural	Urban	Govt. School	Non-Government School
Vikasnagar	-	1	16	11	6	9	8
Sahaspur	-	1	20	10	11	11	10
Raipur	1	2	26	12	17	14	15
Doiwala	1	2	18	12	9	10	11
Total	**2**	**6**	**80**	**45**	**43**	**44**	**44**

(Ref. Appendix-A)

Keeping in view the Gender, Locality and medium of instruction in schools a sample of 800 adolescents studying in XI and XII classes were drawn randomly from the sample inter colleges at the third phase of sample selection. The rural area which fell within the selected developmental blocks was not extreme rural as if fell very much within the periphery of the Urban area.

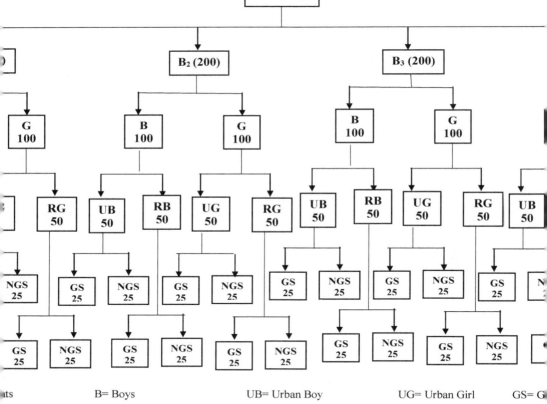

3.5 VARIABLES OF THE STUDY

Independent variable

- Socio-economic status

Dependent Variables

- Self-confidence
- Mental Health
- Personal Values

Socio Demographic independent Variables

- Gender
- Locality
- Type of School

3.6 TOOLS USED

The following tools were used in this research.

- Modified Kuppuswamy scale updated for year 2018(Dr. Sheikh Mohd Saleem)
- Mental Health battery (A.K. Singh and Alpana Singh Gupta)
- Agnihotri self-confidence Inventory (Rekha Gupta)
- Personal values scale (Madhulika Verma/ Vindeshwari Wacar Panwar)

3.6.1 MODIFIED KUPPUSWAMY'S SES SCALE

This scale was devised by Kuppuswamy and is the most widely used scale for determining the socio-economic status of an individual or a family in urban areas. Initially the scale was formulated for determining SES of an individual but later on, it was modified to determine SES of a family rather than and individual. The scale was initially developed by Kuppuswamy in the year 1976 including index parameters like education, occupation, and total income which was further modified in later years to include head of families educational status, occupational status and overall aggregate income of the whole family, pooled from all sources. 8 The Kuppuswamy SES has included 3 parameters and each parameter is further classified into subgroups and scores have been allotted to each subgroup which have been defined later in this paper. The total score of Kuppuswamy SES ranges from 3-29 and it classifies families into 5 groups, "upper class, upper middle class, lower middle class, upper lower and lower socio-economic class." The scale has been revised interminable over the past years because the parameter of overall income of the family from all the sources scale loses its pertinence following the devaluation in the worth of Indian rupee while the occupation of the head of family andeducation of the head of the family remains the same with time.

In order to carry out and perform the regular revision of the scale, the income scale in the Kuppuswamy SES is revised, "as per changes in the consumer price index (CPI) for industrial workers as projected by the central ministry of statistics and programme implementation on their website."9 The values of the CPI are "explicated in reference to a base year". As per the Labour Bureau, Government of India, "the current base year to be taken into account is 2012."10 An update of Kuppuswamy SES 2018 has used the latest base year for calculation purposes and has effectively determined correct income slabs. 11 Here in this paper, we will use 2012 base year for calculating the income level of families to determine their socioeconomic status.

For calculation CPI, the current inflation rate of February 2019 i.e.: 2.57 has been taken into account. 12 If we multiply the generated income scale values of the year 2012 with the conversion factor of 2.57 that will update the Kuppuswamy SES scale for February 2019. 3 The inflation rate is calculated using the formula [(b-a/a) x 100], where 'b' is the CPI of current year and 'a' is the CPI of last year. 13 Kindly refer to Tables 1, 2, 3, and 4 for "Updated Kuppuswamy socioeconomic scale 2019".

Though the Kuppuswamy SES is most widely and favorite scale used by social scientists, researchers in community-based and hospital-based studies. It too has some limitations which render the scales sensitivity in assessing the socioeconomic status of a family. Those include consideration of educational status and type of occupation of the head of the family for calculation of socioeconomic status which is completely unsuitable taking the current scenario into consideration. Moreover, the scale needs the regular scale vulnerable to fluctuations in income levels.

3.6.2 SELF CONFIDENCE INVENTORY

This tool is made by Dr. Rekha Gupta principal of KanoharLal (P.G.) College Meerut (U.P.). The SCI has been designed to assess the level of Self-Confidence among adolescents and adult. The inventory has 56 items.

Reliability: The obtained reliability coefficient and the index of reliability are reported in the following table.

Reliability of the inventory

Method	N	Reliability coefficient	Index of Reliability
Split-Half	362	.91	.95
K-R Formula	200	.89	.94
Test-Retest (After one month)	116	.78	.88

Validity: In the item analysis validity coefficient were determined for each item by bi-serial correlation method and only those items were retained which yielded .25 or above bi-serial correlation with the total score.

The inventory was also validated by correlating the scores obtained on this inventory with the scores obtained by the subject on Basavannas (1975) Self-Confidence Inventory. The validity coefficient obtained is .82 which is significant beyond .01 level.

Instructions for Administration:

1: The inventory is self- administering in nature. In group administration, the instructions, given in the test-booklet may be read aloud by the examiner in order to facilitate starting at a time.

2: There is no fixed time-limit, ordinarily an individual takes 20 minutes to complete the inventory.

Scoring: The inventory can be scored by hand. A score of one is awarded for a response indicative of lack of Self- Confidence, i.e., for making cross to wrong response to item nos. 2, 7, 23, 31, 40, 41, 43, 44, 45, 53, 54, 55 and for making cross to right response to the rest of the item. Hence, the lower the score, the higher would be the level of Self- Confidence and vice-versa.

Norms: The norms have been prepared on a sample of 2074 individuals. Mean, S.D. and Standard Error of means for the total sample are recorded in the given table.

Mean, S.D. and SEM

N	M	S.D.	SE
2074	25.59	10.25	0.22

Norms for interpretation of the level of self-confidence have been given in following table.

Norms for interpretation of the table of self- confidence

Sr. No.	Range of Z-scores	Grade	Level of Self-Confidence
1.	+2.01 and above	A	Extremely Low
2.	+1.26 to +2.00	B	Highly Low
3.	+0.51 to +1.25	C	Above Average Low
4.	-0.50 to +0.50	D	Average
5.	-0.51 to -1.25	E	Above Average
6.	-1.26 to -2.00	F	High
7.	-2.01 and below	G	Extremely high

3.6.3 Personal Value Scale

This scale made by Dr. Madhulika Varma and Vindeswari Waxar Pawar. Dimensions mention in the tool are defined as following:

(I) **Honesty**: Honesty refers to a facet of moral character and denotes positive, virtuous attributes such as integrity, truthfulness and straightforwardness along with absence of lying, cheating and theft.

(II) **Love**: A strong positive emotion of regard and affection based on admiration towards any person and/or object.

(III) **Helpfulness**: the property of providing useful assistance, friendliness evidence by a kindly desposition.

(IV) **Courage**: A quality of moral and mental sprit that enables you to face danger, opposition, or pain without showing fear.

(V) **Good Manners**: The correct way of acting etiquette, being courteous and polite to other, treating all as equals.

(VI) **Faithfulness**: the quality of being loyal, consistent with truth or actuality and doing the right thing for the right person.

(VII) **Discipline**: A systematic method of obtaining obedience, self-control, removal of bad habits and the substitution by good ones and a set of rules regulating behaviors in the right way.

(VIII) **Cleanliness**: The property of being cleanly, good hygiene, neatness of person, place or things. It also includes health, beauty and absence of offensive odor, to avoid the spreading of dirt and contaminants to one self and others.

In this tool there are 50 items. The Dimension-wise distribution of items and their serial number in the scale has been given below.

Dimension-wise serial number of items in the scale

Sr. No.	Dimension	Item wise serial No.							Total items
I	Honesty	13	18	25	31	43	49	-	-	06
II	Love	8	14	26	37	44	46			06
III	Helpfulness	1	5	9	19	27	32	-	-	06
IV	Courage	2	10	20	28	33	38	-	-	06
V	Good manners	6	21	29	34	39	50	-	-	06
VI	Faithfulness	3	11	15	22	30	35	40	45	08
VII	Discipline	12	16	23	36	41	47	-	-	06
VIII	Cleanliness	4	7	17	24	42	48	-	-	06
		Total Number of Items in Scale								50

The scale has no time limit but usually a subject takes 40-50 minutes to finish it. The scale can be administered individually as well as in group. There are 50 items followed by 3 options, they are most desirable, moderate, and least desirable options.

Reliability: Reliability of the personal value scale was established through test-retest method. For establishing the reliability of personal value scale, the scale was administered on 302 students (girls and boys) of CBSE, N. Dehli, to the same student the scale was re-administered at the gap of 20 days. The correlation coefficient was 0.60.

The correlation coefficient were given below.

Test-retest reliability of Personal value scale

	N	Correlation
Test	302	0.606
Re-test	302	

Validity: The content validity of the scale was established by having a discussion with the expert belonging to teachers training institute and schools. Thus the personal value scale was found to be valid.

Directions for Administrations: The personal value scale can be administered individually as well as on a group.

Direction for Scoring: There are 50 items in the scale. The maximum marks should be provided for most valuable condition is 3 and least valuable is 1 and for moderate valuable he score 2 be assigned. For personal value scale maximum obtained scores can be 150, while minimum can be 50.

Personal Value Scale Scoring Key

Sr. No.	Dimensions	Responses Scores		
		a	b	C
1	Helpfulness	1	3	2
2	Courage	1	3	2
3	Faithfulness	3	1	2
4	Cleanliness	1	3	2
5	Helpfulness	2	3	1
6	Good Manners	1	3	2
7	Cleanliness	2	3	1
8	Love	1	3	2
9	Helpfulness	1	2	3

10	Courage	3	1	2
11	Faithfulness	1	2	3
12	Discipline	3	1	2
13	Honesty	2	3	1
14	Love	3	1	2
15	Faithfulness	1	2	3
16	Discipline	1	2	3
17	Cleanliness	1	2	3
18	Honesty	1	3	2
19	Helpfulness	2	3	1
20	Courage	3	2	1
21	Goodmanners	1	3	2
22	Faithfulness	1	3	2
23	Discipline	3	2	1
24	Cleanliness	1	3	2
25	Honesty	1	3	2
26	Love	1	2	3
27	Helpfulness	1	3	2
28	Courage	2	3	1
29	Good manners	2	3	1
30	Faithfulness	1	3	2
31	Honesty	3	1	2
32	Helpfulness	1	2	3
33	Courage	1	1	2
34	Good manners	2	3	1
35	Faithfulness	1	2	3
36	Discipline	2	1	3
37	Love	3	3	2
38	Courage	1	2	3
39	Good manners	2	3	1
40	Faithfulness	1	3	2
41	Discipline	1	3	2
42	Cleanliness	2	3	1
43	Honesty	1	3	2
44	Love	1	3	2
45	Faithfulness	3	2	1
46	Love	2	1	3
47	Discipline	1	2	3
48	Cleanliness	1	3	2
49	Honesty	2	1	3
50	Good manners	3	2	1

Norms:

Norms for interpretation of level of personal values

Sr.No.	Range of z-Scores	Grade	Level of Personal values
1	+2.01 and above	A	Extremely High
2	+1.26 to +2.00	B	High
3	+0.51 to +1.25	C	Above Average
4	-0.50 to +0.50	D	Average
5	-0.51 to -1.25	E	Below Average
6	-1.26 to -2.00	F	Low
7	-2.01 and below	G	Extremely Low

3.6.4 MENTAL HEALTH BATTERY

In the present battery six popular indices of mental health were selected for inclusion.

1: Emotional Stability – It refers to experiencing subjective stability feeling which have positive or negative values for the individual.

2: Over-all Adjustment – It refer to individuals achieving an overall harmonious balance between the demands of various aspects of environment, such as home, health social, emotional and school on the one hand and cognition on the other.

3: Autonomy – It refers to a stage of independence and self-determination in thinking.

4: Security –Insecurity – It refers to a high or low sense of safety, confidence and freedom from fear, apprehension or anxiety particularly with respect to fulfilling the person's present or future needs.

5: Self- concept: It refers to the sum total of the person's attitudes and knowledge towards himself and evaluation of his achievement.

6: Intelligence –It refers to general mental ability which helps the person in thinking rationally, and in behaving purposefully in his environment.

In this battery there are 130 items which are selected dimension wise in the following manner.

Part	Area	Total No. of items
I	Emotional Stability	15
II	Over all Adjustment	40
III	Autonomy	15
IV	Security- Insecurity	15
V	Self-concept	15
VI	Intelligence	30
	TOTAL	130

Instructions

I. Instruction for each part is separate and is printed just before the items. The examinees should read the instruction carefully.

II. There is no time limit for the first five parts.

III. Part VI is a speed test. The total allotted time for this part is 10 minutes.

Scoring

The scoring of Mental Health Battery comprises of two sections-Section A and Section B.

Section A: It determine socio-economic status of the examinee. But in this study the socio-economic status is measeared by Kuppuswamy's SES scale.

Section B: The answers of those items which fully with the answers given in the scoring key would be given a score of +1. If they do not tally, they will be given a score of zero.

Scoring key

PART I	Item Nos.	6,11,13	Yes
	Item Nos.	1,2,3,4,5,7,8,9,10,12,14,15	No
PART II	Item Nos.	16,19,22,26,27,30,35,37,40,41,42,43,47,49,50,52,53	Yes
	Item Nos.	17,18,20,21,23,24,25,28,29,31,32,33,34,36,38,9, 44,45,46,48,51,54,55	No
PART III	Item Nos.	58,60,61,62,63,65,66	Yes
	Item Nos.	56,57,59,64,67,68,69,70	No
PART IV	Item Nos.	71,72,73,74,75,77,79,80,82	Yes
	Item Nos.	76,78,81,83,84.85	No
PART V	Item Nos.	86,87,88,89,91,92,93,94,95,96,97,100	Yes
	Item Nos.	90,98,99	No
PART VI	Item Nos.	101,105,106,109,113,117,125,127	A
	Item Nos.	107,108,110,115,118,119,120,122,123,124,126,129	B
	Item Nos.	103,104,114,121	C
	Item Nos.	102,111,112,116,130	D

Reliability

Both temporal stability reliability and internal consistency reliability of Mental Health Battery were computed.

Reliability coefficient of Mental Health Battery

Part	Area	Mean Age	N	Test-retest reliability	Odd-even (whole length reliability)
I	Emotional Stability	15.6 Yrs.	102	r_{tt}=.876	r_{tt}=.725
II	Over all Adjustment			r_{tt}=.821	r_{tt}=.871
III	Autonomy			r_{tt}=.767	r_{tt}=.812
IV	Security-Insecurity			r_{tt}=826	r_{tt}=.829
V	Self-Concept			r_{tt}=.786	r_{tt}=.861
VI	Intelligence			r_{tt}=.823	r_{tt}=.792

Validity:

Validity Coefficients of Mental Health Battery

parts of Mental Health Battery	N	Concurrent Validity	Parts of Meantal Health Battery	N	Construct Validity
Part I : ES	102	.673*	Part III : AY	102	.681*
Part II : QA		.704*			
Part : IV SI		.821*	Part V : SC		.601*
Part VI : IG		.823*			

Norms

A five point qualitative criterion has been developed for classifying sample with respect to their mental health.

P_{90} and above	Excellent Mental Health
P_{70} to P_{89}	Good Mental Health
P_{50} to P_{69}	Average Mental Health
P_{30} to P_{49}	Poor mental health
Below P_{29}	Very Poor Mental Health

3.7 ADMINISTRATION OF TEST

For the administration of test the researcher in the present study visited personally and contacted directly to the student of XI and XII classes from the selected schools with the permission of Principal and all the four tests were administrated among them at fixed periodic intervals under systematic arrangements.

Following are the important steps undertaken by researcher for the administrating the test:

a. The tests were given to the students one by one and before every test instruction were read loudly by the investigator.
b. There was no fixed time limit for the test but generally 15-20 minutes time was sufficient for completion of one test.
c. It was instructed to the students that they should not consult their friends while answering the questions. He/she is free to ask the investigator, in case of any confusion.
d. As soon as the students completed their task, test material was collected from them.

After data collection the scoring of 800 questionnaires were done according to their scoring procedures.

6.8 STATISTICAL TECHNIQUES USED

After checking the normality of the data, the data was found to be normally distributed therefore parametric statistics is appropriate for the analysis of the data. For the analysis of the data some descriptive and inferential statistics have been used, which are following

- Descriptive statistics such as Mean, Standard Deviation were calculated to describe the nature of data.
- 't' test was used to compare the different groups.
- Pearson Coefficient of Correlation was used to see the relationship between variables.
- ANOVA was used to see the interactional effect.

For the computation and statistical treatment of data, SPSS software was employed with the help of professional analyst.

CHAPTER-IV
ANALYSIS & INTERPRETATION

The next step after collecting the data is of its analysis because the data as such has no meaning unless it is analyzed by the statistical techniques in order to arrive at certain reliable and valid conclusions. This chapter is divided into two main sections, which are

Descriptive statistic- In this section mean and standard deviation have been computed to study and understand all the variables involved in the present study.

Inferential statistics- This section examined the effect of SES on self-confidence, mental health and personal values of adolescents. The relationship between adolescents self-confidence, mental health and personal values was explored and also has been examined the effect of gender, locality and type of school on the self-confidence, mental health and personal values. The data was analyzed by using ANOVA, Pearson coefficient of correlation and 't' test.

PHASE I - To find out the effect of different dimensions of socio-economic status of family on self-confidence of adolescents.

(a) Effect of different dimensions of SES on self-confidence of girl adolescents.

TABLE- 4.1

Mean, Standard Deviation & F Value of Self Confidence of girl adolescents with respect to Socio-Economic Status

Level of SES	N (N=400)	Mean	Std. Deviation	Std. Error	F Value	P Value
lower	2	27.0000	4.24264	3.00000		
lower middle	171	27.6491	9.21027	.70433		
upper	35	20.9429	10.75924	1.81864	4.226	.002
upper lower	79	25.7975	10.35817	1.16539		
upper middle	113	24.7788	8.94999	.84194		

(High mean represent low self-confidence and low mean represent high self-confidence)

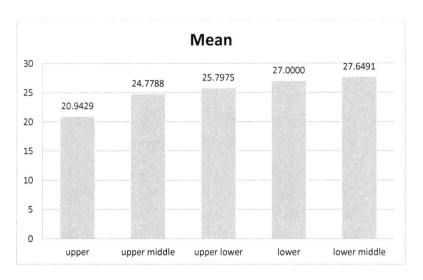

A glance at Table 4.1 clearly reveals that the calculated F value (4.226) is significant at 0.01 level of significance (p<0.01). It means that there exists a significant difference in the self-confidence of Girl adolescents of different socio-economic levels. The above table reveals a significant difference between the mean scores of Lower, Upper lower, Lower Middle, Upper Middle & Upper class subjects. The result further reveals that those girl adolescents who belong to upper class are having high self-confidence than lower class Girl adolescents.

It show that socio-economic status affects the self-confidence of Girl adolescents significantly. It may be that girls in backward classes are not given proper facilities, rights and opportunities for advancement which does not give them an opportunity to develop their personality properly. Which can also cause depression which can be a hindrance in increasing their self-confidence. Whereas in advanced families, girls get equal opportunities for advancement, which may develop their personality and hence they may have better confidence.

(b) Effect of different dimensions of SES on self-confidence of boy adolescents.

TABLE -4.2

Mean, Standard Deviation & F Value of Self Confidence of boy adolescents with respect to Socio-Economic Status

Level of SES	N (N=400)	Mean	Std. Deviation	Std. Error	F value	P value
lower	8	37.0000	7.19126	2.54250	5.560	.000
lower middle	137	25.4015	9.62339	.82218		
upper	27	19.1111	10.77509	2.07367		
upper lower	112	26.0268	10.28728	.97206		
upper middle	116	25.6983	9.91022	.92014		

(High mean represent low self-confidence and low mean represent high self-confidence)

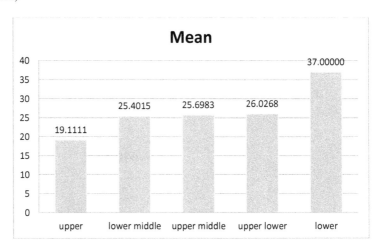

Table 4.2 shows that calculated F value (5.560) is significant at 0.01 level of significance (p<0.01). It means that there exists a significant difference in the self-confidence of Boys adolescents of different socio-economic levels. The above table reveals a significant difference between the mean scores of Lower, Upper lower, Lower Middle, Upper Middle & Upper class subjects. The result further reveals that those Boy adolescents who belong to upper class are having high self-confidence than those

belonging to lower class. It means that we can say with 99% confidence that socio-economic status affects the self-confidence of Boys adolescents significantly.

It may be that boys from backward families do not get adequate educational opportunities as compared to those from advanced families it may hinder their academic achievement. Similar results are reported by **Rather and Sharma (2015)** who revealed that there is an intimate relationship between SES and Academic grades of the students. Academic achievement can affect the self-confidence of adolescents. **Verma, R.K. and Kumari Saroj (2016)** also revealed that significant relationship exists between self-confidence and academic achievement of elementary school students.

(c) Effect of different dimensions of SES on self-confidence of rural girl adolescent.

TABLE-4.3
Mean, Standard Deviation & F Value of Self Confidence of Rural Girl adolescents with respect to Socio-Economic Status

Level of SES	N (N=200)	Mean	Std. Deviation	Std. Error	F Value	P value
lower middle	83	26.2410	8.65827	.95037	3.604	.007
upper	24	18.0417	9.25710	1.88960		
upper lower	38	24.0000	10.93717	1.77424		
upper middle	54	23.7963	9.75237	1.32713		

(High mean represent low self-confidence and low mean represent high self-confidence)

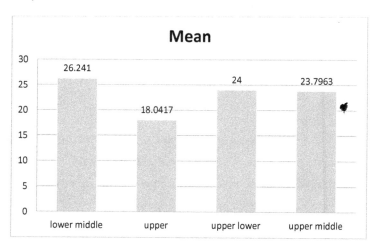

Table 4.3 shows that the calculated F value (3.604) is significant at 0.01 level of significance (p<0.01). It means that there exists a significant difference in the self-confidence of rural Girl adolescents of different socio-economic levels. The above table reveals a significant difference between the mean scores of Lower, Upper lower, Lower Middle, Upper Middle & Upper class subjects. The result further reveals that those Rural Girl adolescents who belong to upper class have high self-confidence as compared to the lower class rural girl adolescents.

It has been observed that self-confidence and socio-economic status of family are positively related to each other. According to **Filippin Antonio & Paccagnella Marco (2011)** which revealed that there is a correlation between family background and self-confidence. Therefore it may be said that SES levels have positive effect on the self-confidence of rural girl adolescent.

(d) Effect of different dimensions of SES on self-confidence of rural boy adolescents.

TABLE-4.4

Mean, Standard Deviation & F Value of Self Confidence of Rural Boy adolescents with respect to Socio-Economic Status

Level of SES	N (N=200)	Mean	Std. Deviation	Std. Error	F Value	P value
lower	7	37.5714	7.56873	2.86071		
lower middle	75	24.8000	9.52238	1.09955		
upper	13	24.0769	12.58611	3.49076	2.724	.031
upper lower	44	25.7273	10.67569	1.60942		
upper middle	61	25.6885	9.57521	1.22598		

(High mean represent low self-confidence and low mean represent high self-confidence)

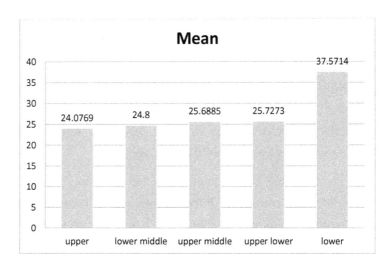

The perusal of table 4.4reveals that calculated F value (2.724) is significant at 0.05 level of significance (p<0.05). It means that there exists a significant difference in the self-confidence of rural Boys adolescents of different socio-economic levels. The above table reveals a significant difference between the mean scores of Lower, Upper lower, Lower Middle, Upper Middle & Upper class subjects. The result further reveals that those Rural Boy adolescents who belong to upper class are having high self-confidence than lower class rural boy adolescents.

It means that we can say with 95% confidence that socio-economic status affects the self-confidence of rural girl adolescents. It may be that the rural areas in Dehradun district are very close to urban areas. Like the urban area, there are people of different SES in the rural area. Therefore in rural areas also the high SES families provides the proper awareness, technological impact, motivation etc. to the boy adolescents to meet their basic needs which boosts their self-confidence. On the other hand, families with low socio-economic status do not meet the needs of boy adolescents which can lower their self-confidence. So the self-confidence of rural boy adolescents is different because of the SES of their family.

(e) Effect of different dimensions of SES on self-confidence of urban girl adolescents.

TABLE-4.5

Mean, Standard Deviation & F Value of Self Confidence of Urban Girl adolescents with respect to Socio-Economic Status

Level of SES	N (N=200)	Mean	Std. Deviation	Std. Error	F Value	P value
lower middle	88	28.9773	9.56163	1.01927		
upper	11	27.2727	11.49862	3.46696		
upper lower	41	27.4634	9.62574	1.50329	1.159	.330
upper middle	59	25.6780	8.12710	1.05806		

(High mean represent low self-confidence and low mean represent high self-confidence)

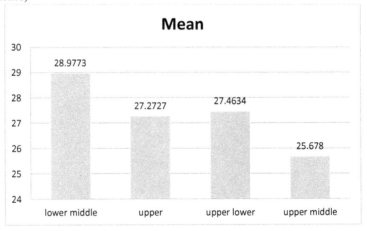

From the content of the table 4.5 it is revealed that the calculated F value (1.159) is not significant at 0.05 level of significance (p>0.05). It means that there exists no significant difference in the self-confidence of Urban Girls adolescents of different socio-economic levels.

People with any socio-economic status in urban areas try to maintain their status in society. They create a healthy environment in the family. Urban families exposes adolescents to new world views, technologies and life styles. So the girls in urban areas get lot of opportunities in their families and school for their successful growth and development. Success and achievement help them to feel good about themselves which may promote self-confidence in them.

(f) Effect of different dimensions of SES on self-confidence of urban boy adolescents.

TABLE-4.6

Mean, Standard Deviation & F Value of Self Confidence of Urban Boy adolescents with respect to Socio-Economic Status

Level of SES	N (N=200)	Mean	Std. Deviation	Std. Error	F Value	P value
lower middle	62	26.1290	9.77196	1.24104		
upper	14	14.5000	6.19864	1.65665		
upper lower	68	26.2206	10.10371	1.22525	4.633	.001
upper middle	55	25.7091	10.35781	1.39665		

(High mean represent low self-confidence and low mean represent high self-Confidence)

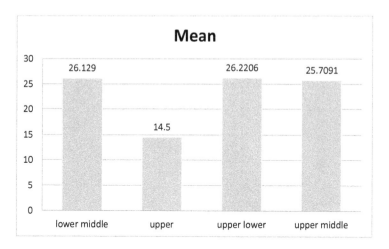

A glance at table 4.6 clearly reveals that the calculated F value (4.633) is significant at 0.01 level of significance (p<0.01). It means that there exists a significant difference in the self-confidence of urban boy adolescents of different socio-economic levels. The above table reveals a significant difference between the mean scores of Lower, Upper lower, Lower Middle, Upper Middle & Upper class subjects. The result further reveals that those urban boy adolescents who belong to upper class are having high self-confidence than those who belong to lower classes. Thus we can say with 99% confidence that SES of urban boy adolescents affect their self-confidence.

Wankhade and Rokade (2011) revealed that the self-confidence of male and female from urban areas found almost same. This means that the area has no effect on the adolescent's self-confidence. But since socio-economic status is responsible for self-confidence therefore the self-confidence of urban boy adolescents of differs with different SES.

(g) Effect of different dimensions of SES on self-confidence of girl adolescents from government school.

TABLE-4.7

Mean, Standard Deviation & F Value of Self Confidence of Girls from Government school with respect to Socio-Economic Status

Level of SES	N (N=200)	Mean	Std. Deviation	Std. Error	F Value	P value
lower	2	27.0000	4.24264	3.00000	1.112	.352
lower middle	114	27.6930	9.55017	.89446		
upper lower	71	26.4930	10.59902	1.25787		
upper middle	12	28.2500	11.00516	3.17692		

(High mean represent low self-confidence and low mean represent high self-confidence)

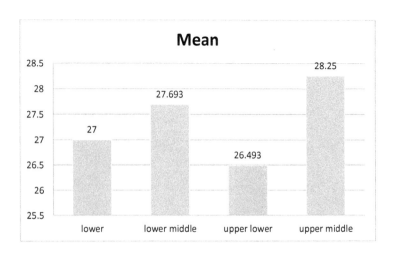

A perusal of table 4.7 reveals that the calculated F value (1.112) is not significant at 0.05 level of significance (p>0.05). It means that there exists no significant difference in the self-confidence of Government School Girl adolescents of different socio-economic levels. Its shows that socio-economic status does not affect the self-confidence of Government School Girl adolescents.

It may be that the maximum girl adolescents studying in government schools, as shown in the table 4.7, belong to lower middle and upper lower SES families in comparison to upper SES families. Therefore it may be due to low difference in their socio-economic level, there is no difference in their self-confidence also.

(h) Effect of different dimensions of SES on self-confidence of boy adolescents from government school.

TABLE-4.8
Mean, Standard Deviation & F Value of Self Confidence of Boy adolescents from Government school with respect to Socio-Economic Status

Level of SES	N (N=200)	Mean	Std. Deviation	Std. Error	F Value	P value
lower	8	37.0000	7.19126	2.54250	4.667	.001
lower middle	76	25.1447	10.38422	1.19115		
upper lower	103	26.4660	10.46639	1.03128		
upper middle	12	20.8333	7.70871	2.22531		

High mean represent low self-confidence and low mean represent high self-confidence)

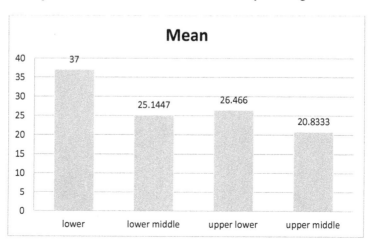

A perusal of table 4.8reveals that the statistically calculated F value (4.667) is significant at 0.01 level of significance (p<0.01). It means that there exists a significant difference in the self-confidence of Government School boy adolescents of different socio-economic levels. The above table reveals a significant difference between the mean scores of Lower, Upper lower, Lower Middle, Upper Middle & Upper class subjects. The result further reveals that those Government School boy adolescent who belong to upper class are having high self-confidence than lower class Government School boy adolescents.

It may be that families with high SES provide more facilities to boy adolescent regardless of the type of school they may go to. Whereas families with lower socio-economic status are unable provide them facilities due to lack of money. Which makes a difference in the self-confidence of boy even while studying in the same school. Therefore we are 99% confident that the SES of families affect self-confidence of the boy adolescent studying in government school.

(i) **Effect of different dimensions of SES on self -confidence of Girl adolescents from non -government school.**

TABLE-4.9

Mean, Standard Deviation & F Value of Self Confidence of Girl adolescents from Non-Government school with respect to Socio-Economic Status

Level of SES	N (N=200)	Mean	Std. Deviation	Std. Error	F Value	P value
lower middle	57	27.5614	8.57117	1.13528	4.497	.004
upper	34	21.3235	10.67912	1.83145		
upper lower	8	19.6250	4.86790	1.72106		
upper middle	101	24.3663	8.64722	.86043		

(High mean represent low self-confidence and low mean represent high self-confidence)

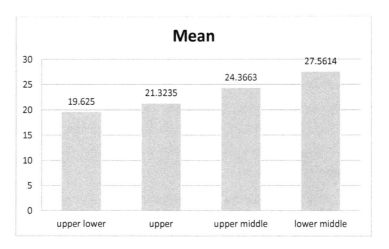

Table 4.9 shows that the calculated F value (4.497) is significant at 0.01 level of significance (p<0.01). It means that there exists a significant difference in the self-confidence of Non-Government School Girl adolescents of different socio-economic levels. The above table reveals a significant difference between the mean scores of Lower, Upper lower, Lower Middle, Upper Middle & Upper class subjects. The result further reveals that those girl adolescents studying in Non-government schools and belonging to upper class are having high self-confidence as compared to those belonging lower class Non-Government School Girl adolescents.

It may be because in Indian society girl spend, most of their times with in a family. They are more close to their parents. They get inspiration from their parents. Therefore the environment of the family affects their behavior. The socio-economic level of the family has an impact on the home environment also. **Barnad, Bee Hammond and Siegel (1984)** also agree with this stating that there is a positive relationship between SES and home environment. They found that the children belonging to families of higher socio-economic classes received more beneficial home environment. Result of **Denga (1986)** opined that home environment to a great extent, influences the child's behavior and achievement. The achievement of the adolescents is related with their self-confidence. According to **Fareen Fatma (2015)** there is a positive correlation between self-confidence and academic achievement of adolescents. Therefore we can say with 99% confidence that the self-confidence of girl adolescents is affected by socio-economic status of their family.

(j) Effect of different dimensions of SES on self-confidence of boy adolescents from non-government school.

TABLE-4.10

Mean, Standard Deviation & F Value of Self Confidence of Boy adolescents from Non-Government school with respect to Socio-Economic Status

Level of SES	N (N=200)	Mean	Std. Deviation	Std. Error	F Value	P value
lower middle	61	25.7213	8.65666	1.10837	3.848	.010
upper	26	19.7692	10.42039	2.04361		
upper lower	9	21.0000	6.38357	2.12786		
upper middle	104	26.2596	10.01164	.98172		

(High mean represent low self-confidence and low mean represent high self-confidence)

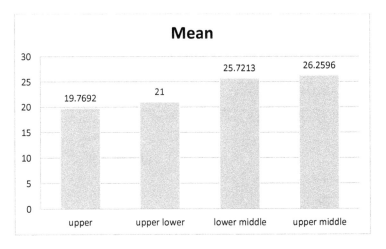

The perusal of table 4.10 reveals that the calculated F value (3.848) is significant at 0.01 level of significance ($p<0.01$). It means that there exists a significant difference in the self-confidence of Non-Government School boy adolescents of different socio-economic levels. The above table reveals a significant difference between the mean scores of Lower, Upper lower, Lower Middle, Upper Middle & Upper class subjects. The result further reveals that those Non-Government School boy adolescents who belong to upper class are having high self-confidence than lower class Non-Government School boy adolescents.

It may be inferred that home environment is responsible for self-confidence. And because the socio-economic level of the family has an influence on the home environment **(Barnad, Bee Hammond and Siegel, 1984).** Therefore the self-confidence of boy adolescents is also affected by the socio-economic status of family.

(k) Effect of different dimensions of SES on self -confidence of adolescents.

TABLE- 4.11
Mean, Standard Deviation & F Value of Self-Confidence of adolescents with respect to Socio-Economic Status

Level of SES	N (N= 800).	Mean	Std. Deviation	Std. Error	F Value	P Value
Lower	10	35.0000	7.74597	2.44949	8.208	.000
lower middle	308	26.6494	9.44729	.53831		
Upper	62	20.1452	10.71669	1.36102		
upper lower	191	25.9319	10.29003	.74456		
upper middle	229	25.2445	9.43916	.62376		

(High mean represent low self-confidence and low mean represent high self-confidence)

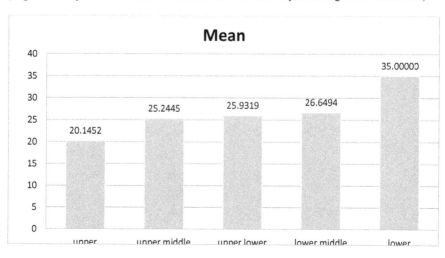

The perusal of Table 4.11 reveals that calculated F value (8.208) is significant at 0.01 level of significance (p<0.01). It means that there exists a significant difference in the self-confidence of adolescents of different socio-economic levels. The above table reveals a significant difference between the mean scores of Lower, Upper lower, Lower Middle, Upper Middle & Upper class categories of SES scales. The result further reveals that those adolescents who belong to upper class are having high self-confidence than lower class SES adolescents. Here we are 99% confident that SES affects Self-confident of adolescents. It shows that socio-economic status affect the self-confidence of adolescents significantly.

It may be that the socio-economic status of adolescents from difficult background may have difficulty in accessing basic needs and this may interfere with the attainment of positive self-confidence in them. Those adolescents from advanced background will have their basic needs met and therefore have a better chance of attaining a positive self-confidence. The result is consistent with the study made by **Filippin Antonio & Paccagnella Marco (2011)** which revealed that there is a correlation between family background and self-confidence.

Hence, in Phase-I we observed that in most of the cases the result was found to be significantly different. Therefore, the hypothesis I stating **"There exists no significant difference between different dimensions of socio-economic status and self-confidence of adolescents"** is partially rejected.

PHASE II- To find the effect of different dimensions of socio-economic status of family on mental health of adolescents.

a) **Effect of different dimensions of SES on mental health of girl adolescents.**

TABLE-4.12

Mean, Standard Deviation & F Value of Mental Health of Girl Adolescents with respect to Socio-Economic Status

Level of SES	Number of adolescents	Mean	Std. Deviation	Std. Error	F value	P value
Lower	2	74.5000	.70711	.50000		
lower middle	171	75.7427	9.20507	.70393		

Upper	35	76.5714	9.36918	1.58368	4.984	.00
upper lower	79	79.5823	8.86596	.99750		
upper middle	113	73.7522	8.67007	.81561		

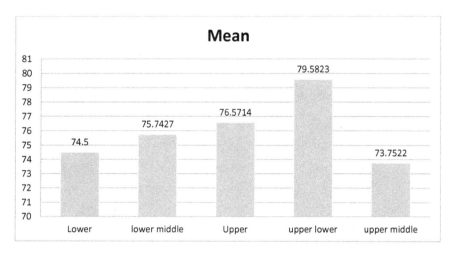

A perusal of table 4.12reveals that calculated F value (4.984) which is significant at 0.01 level of significance (p<0.01). It means that there exists a significant difference in the Mental Health of Girl adolescents of different socio-economic levels. The above table reveals a significant difference between the mean scores of Lower, Upper lower, Lower Middle, Upper Middle & Upper class subjects. The result further reveals that those Girl adolescents who belong to upper classes are having high Mental Health than those belonging to lower classes. Its show that socio-economic status affects the Mental Health of Girls adolescents.

This may be because there is a positive relationship between the socio-economic status of family and the home environment **(Barnad, Bee Hammond and Siegal, 1984)** and girls are more in touch with their family. Therefore the home environment affect their mental health more. The study made by **Manguvani E (1990)** is in congruence with this statement. She found that the home environment is significant contributor to all components of mental health.

b) **Effect of different dimensions of SES on mental health of boy adolescent.**

TABLE-4.13

Mean, Standard Deviation & F Value of Mental Health of Boy Adolescents with respect to Socio-Economic Status

Level of SES	Number of adolescents	Mean	Std. Deviation	Std. Error	F value	P value
Lower	8	70.2500	4.55914	1.61190		
lower middle	137	75.0657	11.27543	.96333		
Upper	27	76.7778	13.00394	2.50261	.768	.547
upper lower	112	75.5536	10.60498	1.00208		
upper middle	116	74.3621	9.51374	.88333		

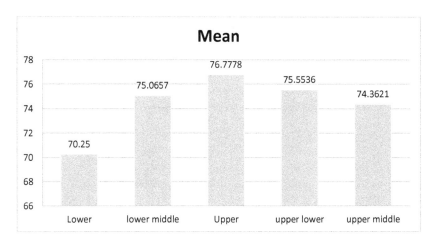

A careful inspection of Table 4.13 reveals that calculated F value (.768) is not significant at 0.05 level of significance (p>0.05). It means that there exists no significant difference in the Mental Health of Boy adolescents of different socio-economic levels. It shows that socio-economic status does not affect the Mental Health of Boy adolescents.

It may be that the environment affects the boy adolescents more than the SES of his family. In this modern time, social media is playing very important role in shaping the life style of boy adolescents. This create some behavioral problems like aggression, frustration, antisocial behavior etc. in them which affect their mental health. The study made by **Chakravorty and Srivastava (2002)** is in congruence with this statement. They studied that aggressiveness in adolescents significantly and positively associated with using media. Therefore in the context of boy adolescents, we can say that the mental health of boy adolescents is not affected by the SES of family but may be by the present social environment.

c) **Effect of different dimensions of SES on mental health of rural girl.**

TABLE-4.14

Mean, Standard Deviation & F Value of Mental Health of Rural Girl Adolescents with respect to Socio-Economic Status

Level of SES	Number of adolescents	Mean	Std. Deviation	Std. Error	F value	P value
lower middle	83	76.7711	8.51158	.93427		
Upper	24	78.6667	9.62635	1.96497		
upper lower	38	80.1316	10.48595	1.70105	1.985	.098
upper middle	54	75.0741	8.27328	1.12585		

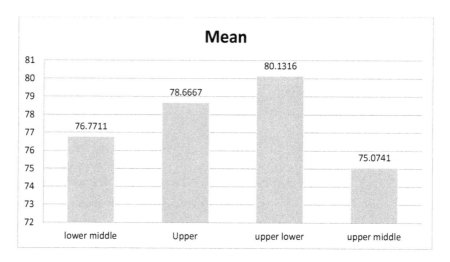

A glance of table 4.14 clearly reveals that the calculated F value (1.985) is not significant at 0.05 level of significance (p>0.05). It means that there exists no significant difference in the Mental Health of Rural Girl adolescents of different socio-economic levels. Its show that socio-economic status not affect the Mental Health of Rural Girl adolescents.

It may be that in rural areas all people live in harmony with each other. There is a feeling of brotherhood among them. Despite different SES the families give healthy environment to their children. Due to which the environment of the rural area remains healthy and because girls are more in touch with their family. Hence the SES of the family has no effect on the mental health of girl adolescent due to the healthy environment in all the families in rural areas.

d) **Effect of different dimensions of SES on mental health of total rural boy adolescents.**

TABLE-4.15

Mean, Standard Deviation & F Value of Mental Health of Rural Boy Adolescents with respect to Socio-Economic Status

Level of SES	Number of adolescents	Mean	Std. Deviation	Std. Error	F value	P value
Lower	7	70.7143	4.71573	1.78238	.403	.807
lower middle	75	74.6667	11.57856	1.33698		
Upper	13	73.9231	13.18118	3.65580		
upper lower	44	75.7727	10.30661	1.55378		
upper middle	61	74.2787	9.07218	1.16157		

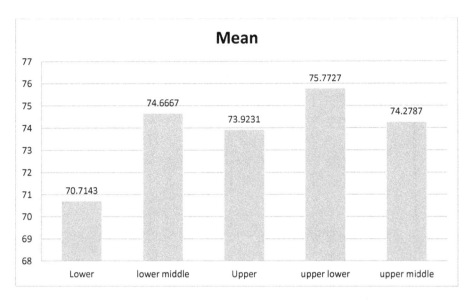

A careful inspection of table 4.15 reveals that the calculated F value (.403) is not significant at 0.05 level of significance (p>0.05). It means that there exists a no significant difference in the Mental Health of Rural Boy adolescents of different socio-economic levels. It shows that socio-economic status does not affect the Mental Health of Rural Boy adolescents.

It may also be that in Indian society boys are given more advantage then girls irrespective of the SES of family. The boys are mostly affected more by social environment than the family because the adolescent boys give more importance to society and peers and the social environment affects their mental health accordingly. The study made by **Mittal, A (2008)** is in congruence with these statement. He found that the mental health of students of different localities is significant. It may be that the overall social environment in rural areas is healthy therefore, boy adolescents have same mental health regardless of the SES of their families. Therefore, due to the positive environment in rural areas, the SES of the family of boy adolescents has no effect on their mental health.

e) **Effect of different dimensions of SES on mental health of urban girl adolescents.**

TABLE-4.16

Mean, Standard Deviation & F Value of Mental Health of Urban Girl Adolescents with respect to Socio-Economic Status

Level of SES	Number of adolescents	Mean	Std. Deviation	Std. Error	F value	P value
lower middle	88	74.7727	9.76356	1.04080		
Upper	11	72.0000	7.19722	2.17004		
upper lower	41	79.0732	7.14279	1.11552	3.581	.008
upper middle	59	72.5424	8.91593	1.16076		

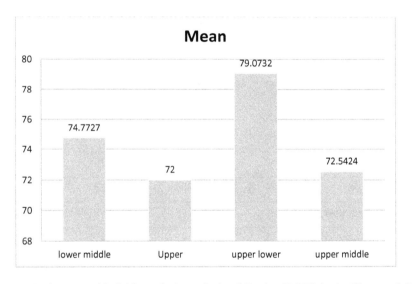

A glance at table 4.16 reveals that calculated F value (3.581) is significant at 0.01 level of significance (p<0.01). It means that there exists a significant difference in the Mental Health of Urban Girl adolescents of different socio-economic levels. The above table reveals a significant difference between the mean scores of Lower, Upper lower, Lower Middle, Upper Middle & Upper class subjects. The result further reveals that those Urban Girl adolescents who belong to upper classes are having high Mental Health than those belonging to lower classes. Here we are 99% confident to say that socio-economic status affects the Mental Health of Urban Girls adolescents.

It may be that people living in urban areas are influenced by its pomp & show. In such a situation urban girls also have a lot of desires and dreams. These desires of girls from high SES are easily met whereas due to lake of money in families with low

SES, they are unable to fulfill their desires which can cause stress condition in them, which can affect their mental health. Hence the SES of the family in urban areas affect the mental health of the girl adolescent.

f) **Effect of different dimensions of SES on mental health of urban boy adolescents.**

TABLE-4.17

Mean, Standard Deviation & F Value of Mental Health of Urban Boy Adolescents with respect to Socio-Economic Status

Level of SES	Number of adolescents	Mean	Std. Deviation	Std. Error	F value	P value
lower middle	62	75.5484	10.97191	1.39343	.743	.564
Upper	14	79.4286	12.73224	3.40283		
upper lower	68	75.4118	10.86722	1.31784		
upper middle	55	74.4545	10.06427	1.35707		

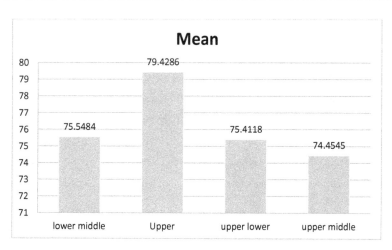

A perusal of table 4.17reveals that the calculated F value (.403) is non-significant at 0.05 level of significance (p>0.05). It means that there exists no significant difference in the Mental Health of Urban Boy adolescents of different socio-economic levels. It shows that socio-economic status does not affect the Mental Health of Urban Boys adolescents.

As we know adolescent boys have a greater effect of social environment on them than their family. It may happen that teenagers in urban areas develop bad habits like drugs, smoking, drinking etc. Which affect their mental health adversely. Therefore in the urban areas the mental health of boy adolescent is not affected by the socio economic status of their family.

g) **Effect of different dimensions of SES on mental health of government school girl adolescents.**

TABLE-4.18

Mean, Standard Deviation & F Value of Mental Health of Government School girl Adolescents with respect to Socio-Economic Status

Level of SES	Number of adolescents	Mean	Std. Deviation	Std. Error	F value	P value
Lower	2	74.5000	.70711	.50000		
lower middle	114	76.5263	9.25376	.86669		
upper lower	71	79.5211	9.17739	1.08916	1.990	.098
upper middle	12	74.8333	10.30299	2.97422		

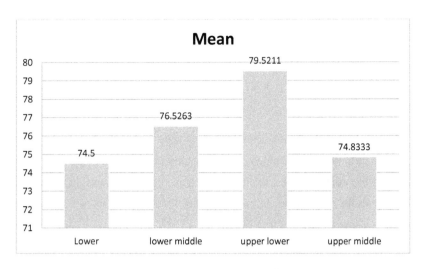

The study of table 4.18 reveals that the calculated F value (1.990) is not significant at 0.05 level of significance (p>0.05). It means that there exists a no significant difference in the Mental Health of Government School Girl adolescents of different socio-economic levels. It shows that socio-economic status does not affect the Mental Health of Government School Girl adolescents.

Table 4.18 also reveals that out of 200 girl adolescents, 114 belong to lower middle SES families. And because due to the same SES their mental health is also similar. Therefore no difference has been found in the mental health of the girl adolescents studying in government schools.

h) **Effect of different dimensions of SES on mental health of government school boy adolescents.**

TABLE-4.19

Mean, Standard Deviation & F Value of Mental Health of Government School boy Adolescents with respect to Socio-Economic Status

Level of SES	Number of adolescents	Mean	Std. Deviation	Std. Error	F value	P value
Lower	8	70.2500	4.55914	1.61190		
lower middle	76	75.3816	12.72474	1.45963		
upper lower	103	76.0097	10.53891	1.03843	2.254	.065
upper middle	12	82.0000	8.11284	2.34198		

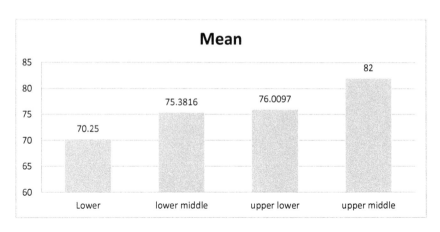

From the contents of Table 4.19 it is revealed that the calculated F value (2.254) is not significant at 0.05 level of significance (p>0.05). It means that there exists a no significant difference in the Mental Health of Government School Boys adolescents of different socio-economic levels. Its shows that socio-economic status does not affect the Mental Health of Government School Boy adolescents. This may be because no difference was found in the mental health of boys studying in the same school environment.

i) **Effect of different dimensions of SES on mental health of non -government school girl adolescents.**

TABLE-4.20

Mean, Standard Deviation & F Value of Mental Health of Non-Government School girl Adolescents with respect to Socio-Economic Status

Level of SES	Number of adolescents	Mean	Std. Deviation	Std. Error	F value	P value
lower middle	57	74.1754	8.98237	1.18974	1.898	.131
Upper	34	76.1471	9.16228	1.57132		
upper lower	8	80.1250	5.76783	2.03924		
upper middle	101	73.6238	8.50629	.84641		

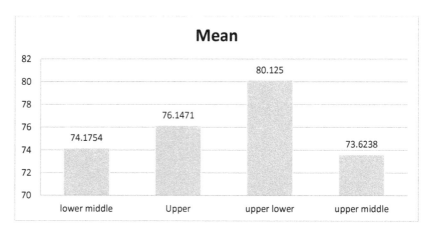

A careful inspection of table 4.20 reveals that the calculated F value (1.898) is not significant at 0.05 level of significance (p>0.05). It means that there exists a no significant difference in the Mental Health of Non-Government School Girl adolescents of different socio-economic levels. It shows that socio-economic status does not affect the Mental Health of Non-Government School Girls adolescents.

Adolescence is an important period for developing and maintaining social and emotional habits for good mental health. Supporting environment in the family and at school are also important. Adolescents studying in non-government school may also have good environment, therefore they may have similar mental health due to studying in the similar school environment.

j) Effect of different dimensions of SES on mental health of non- government school boy adolescents.

TABLE-4.21

Mean, Standard Deviation & F Value of Mental Health of Non-Government School boy Adolescents with respect to Socio-Economic Status

Level of SES	Number of adolescents	Mean	Std. Deviation	Std. Error	F value	P value
lower middle	61	74.6721	9.24612	1.18384		
Upper	26	76.0385	12.66959	2.48471		
upper lower	9	70.3333	10.53565	3.51188	.981	.403

| upper middle | 104 | 73.4808 | 9.29765 | .91171 | | |

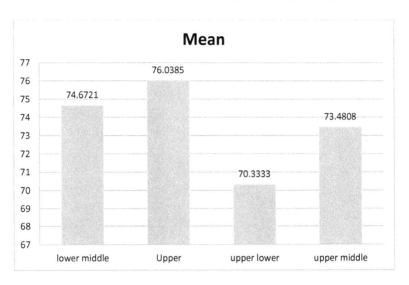

A glance at table 4.21 clearly reveals that the calculated F value (.981) is not significant at 0.05 level of significance (p>0.05). It means that there exist a no significant difference in the Mental Health of Non-Government School Boy adolescents of different socio-economic levels. It shows that socio-economic status does not affect the Mental Health of Non-Government School Boys adolescents.

This could be because there is no difference in the mental health of boys from non-government school due to studying in the same school environment.

k) **Effect of different dimensions of SES on mental health of adolescents.**

TABLE-4.22

Mean, Standard Deviation & F Value of Mental Health of Adolescents with respect to Socio-Economic Status

Level of SES	Number of adolescents	Mean	Std. Deviation	Std. Error	F value	P value
Lower	10	71.1000	4.40833	1.39403		
lower middle	308	75.4416	10.16636	.57928		
Upper	62	76.6613	11.00066	1.39709	3.378	.009

| upper lower | 191 | 77.2199 | 10.09606 | .73052 | | |
| upper middle | 229 | 74.0611 | 9.09240 | .60084 | | |

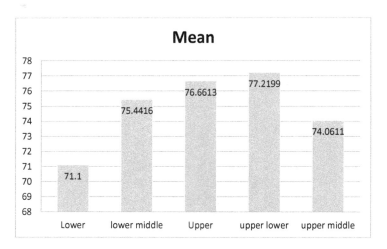

The statistically calculated F value (3.378) is significant at 0.01 level of significance (p<0.01). It means that there exist a significant difference in the Mental Health of adolescents of different socio-economic levels. The above table reveals a significant difference between the mean scores of Lower, Upper lower, Lower Middle, Upper Middle & Upper class subjects. The result further reveals that those adolescents who belong to upper class are having high Mental Health than those from the lower class. It is inferred from this that socio-economic status affects the Mental Health of adolescents significantly.

It may mean that if SES of family is high then Mental Health of adolescent is also high and vice-versa. The result is consistent with the study made by **Rai and Yadav (1993)** which revealed that Mental Health of low socio-economic status students is lower than that of the Students of higher socio-economic status. Another study made by **Ebong (2004)** also stand in congruence with the above finding. It is found that the children of higher socio-economic group tend to be more creative and intellectually sound than those of the lower and middle groups.

Hence in phase-II, we observed that in most of the cases the result was found to be non-significant difference. But in totality there exists a significant difference in the mental health of adolescents of difference socio-economic status. Thus the II Hypothesis predicting that **"There exists no significant difference of different dimensions of socio-economic status on mental health of adolescents"** is partially rejected.

PHASE III- To find the effect of different dimensions of socio-economic status of family on personal values of adolescents.

a) **Effect of different dimensions of SES on personal values of girl adolescents.**

TABLE-4.23

Mean, Standard Deviation & F Value of Personal Values of Adolescents with respect to Socio-Economic Status

Level of SES	Number of adolescents	Mean	Std. Deviation	Std. Error	F value	P value
Lower	2	114.5000	13.43503	9.50000		
lower middle	171	133.4386	15.00747	1.14765		
Upper	35	135.9143	16.77423	2.83536	5.678	.000
upper lower	79	138.9241	13.11759	1.47584		
upper middle	113	129.8584	13.70080	1.28886		

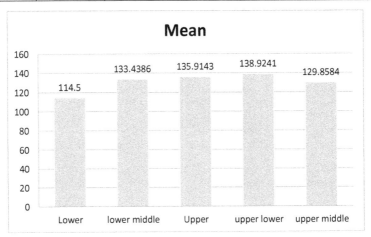

The perusal of table 4.23 reveals that the calculated F value (5.678) is significant at 0.01 level of significance ($p<0.01$). It means that there exists a significant difference in the personal values of girl adolescents of different socio-economic levels. The above table reveals a significant difference between the mean scores of Lower, Upper lower, Lower Middle, Upper Middle & Upper class subjects. The result further reveals that those girl adolescents who belong to upper classes are having high personal values than the lower class girl adolescents. Here we are 99% confident that the SES affects the personal values of girl adolescents.

The reason for this may be that girls are more in touch with their families. The family environment has a direct effect on them and because the education, income and occupation of the parents of adolescents with low SES, all three are of low standard. That is why the home-environment can also be low, which may affect the personal values of girl adolescents. Whereas parents from higher SES are more educated and they try to inculcate good values in their children. **Blais (2010)** also found that personal values will be developed through being influenced by family, culture, society, environment, religious believe and ethnicity. Therefor differences have been found in the person values of girls of different SES families.

b) **Effect of different dimensions of SES on personal values of boy adolescents.**

TABLE-4.24

Mean, Standard Deviation & F Value of Personal Values of Adolescents with respect to Socio-Economic Status

Level of SES	Number of adolescents	Mean	Std. Deviation	Std. Error	F value	P valu
Lower	8	119.3750	12.01116	4.24658		
lower middle	137	129.8540	18.73913	1.60099		
Upper	27	133.5926	19.69041	3.78942	2.729	.0
upper lower	112	134.7143	17.64843	1.66762		
upper middle	116	129.3879	14.85628	1.37937		

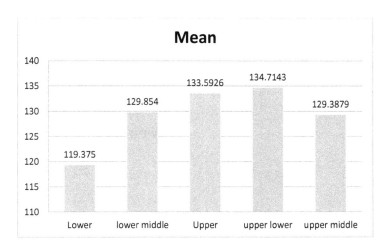

From the content of the table 4.24 it is revealed that the calculated F value (2.729) is significant at 0.05 level of significance ($p<0.05$). It means that there exist a significant difference in the personal values of boy adolescents of different socio-economic levels. The above table reveals a significant difference between the mean scores of Lower, Upper lower, Lower Middle, Upper Middle & Upper class subjects. The result further reveals that those boy adolescents who belong to upper classes are having high personal values than the lower class boy adolescents. It shows that socio-economic status affect the Personal Values of boy adolescents.

It may be that boys from backward families do not get adequate educational opportunities as compared to those from advanced families which may create academic dissatisfaction among them. **Gupta (1992)** found that academic satisfaction was significantly related to their personality need and values. Therefor boys from high SES families have better personal values than boys from lower SES families.

c) **Effect of different dimensions of SES on personal values of rural girl adolescents.**

TABLE-4.25

Mean, Standard Deviation & F Value of Personal Values of Adolescents with respect to Socio-Economic Status

Level of SES	Number of adolescents	Mean	Std. Deviation	Std. Error	F value	P value
lower middle	83	135.9880	15.73833	1.72751		

Upper	24	140.7083	15.02600	3.06717	2.859	.02
upper lower	38	139.6053	14.73099	2.38968		
upper middle	54	132.8704	13.15086	1.78961		

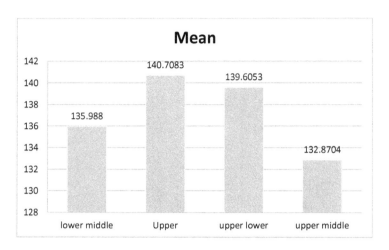

Table 4.25 shows that calculated F value (2.859) is significant at 0.05 level of significance (p<0.05). It means that there exist a significant difference in the personal values of rural girl adolescents of different socio-economic levels. The above table reveals a significant difference between the mean scores of Lower, Upper lower, Lower Middle, Upper Middle & Upper class subjects. The result further reveals that those rural girl adolescents who belong to upper classes are having high personal values than the lower class rural girl adolescents. It mean that socio-economic status affect the Personal Values of rural girl adolescents.

The reason of this may be that the rural areas of Dehradun district are semi urban. In rural areas as well in urban areas, there is a difference in the SES of families. **Nagrajan, P. et. al. (2020)** revealed that the family income plays a crucial role in the personal values of adolescents. Therefore, variation has been found in the personal values of girl adolescents of different SES of rural areas.

d) **Effect of different dimensions of SES on personal values of rural boy adolescents.**

TABLE-4.26
Mean, Standard Deviation & F Value of Personal Values of Adolescents with respect to Socio-Economic Status

Level of SES	Number of adolescents	Mean	Std. Deviation	Std. Error	F value	P value
Lower	7	116.4286	9.34268	3.53120		
lower middle	75	129.7733	19.09901	2.20536		
Upper	13	127.9231	20.48764	5.68225	2.466	.046
upper lower	44	135.6818	16.65487	2.51082		
upper middle	61	128.2295	15.30511	1.95962		

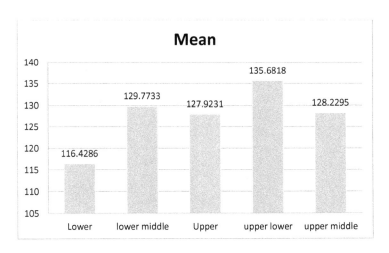

A glance at Table 4.26 clearly reveals that the calculated F value (2.466) is significant at 0.05 level of significance (p<0.05). It means that there exist a significant difference in the personal values of rural boy adolescents of different socio-economic levels. The above table reveals a significant difference between the mean scores of Lower, Upper lower, Lower Middle, Upper Middle & Upper class subjects. The result further reveals that those rural boy adolescents who belong to upper classes are having high personal values than the lower class rural boy adolescents. Thus we can say with 95% confidence that socio-economic status of rural boy affect their Personal Values. **Robert REL, Bengtson VL. (1999)** stated that families are an important factor for the development children's values. That is why the personal values of boys in rural areas are difference due to different SES.

e) **Effect of different dimensions of SES on personal values of urban girl adolescents.**

TABLE-4.27

Mean, Standard Deviation & F Value of Personal Values of Adolescents with respect to Socio-Economic Status

Level of SES	Number of adolescents	Mean	Std. Deviation	Std. Error	F value	P value
lower middle	88	131.0341	13.94937	1.48701	4.714	.00
Upper	11	125.4545	16.18248	4.87920		
upper lower	41	138.2927	11.57420	1.80759		
upper middle	59	127.1017	13.72098	1.78632		

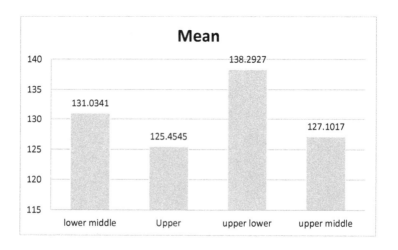

A careful inspection of Table 4.27 reveals that the calculated F value (4.714) is significant at 0.01 level of significance (p<0.01). It means that there exist a significant difference in the personal values of urban girl adolescents of different socio-economic levels. The above table reveals a significant difference between the mean scores of Lower, Upper lower, Lower Middle, Upper Middle & Upper class subjects. The result further reveals that those urban girl adolescents who belong to upper classes are having high personal values than the lower class urban girl adolescents. It shows that socio-economic status affect the Personal Values of urban girl adolescents.

The reason for this may be that education is very expensive in the urban areas of Dehradun district. Only adolescents with high SES are able to take admission in higher standard school. Whereas families with low SES are unable to get their children admitted in these schools due to lack of money. Due to which educational dissatisfaction may arise in them.

f) **Effect of different dimensions of SES on personal values of urban boy adolescents.**

TABLE-4.28

Mean, Standard Deviation & F Value of Personal Values of Adolescents with respect to Socio-Economic Status

Level of SES	Number of adolescents	Mean	Std. Deviation	Std. Error	F value	P value
lower middle	62	129.9516	18.44925	2.34306	1.133	.342
Upper	14	138.8571	18.05486	4.82536		
upper lower	68	134.0882	18.35694	2.22611		
upper middle	55	130.6727	14.37211	1.93794		

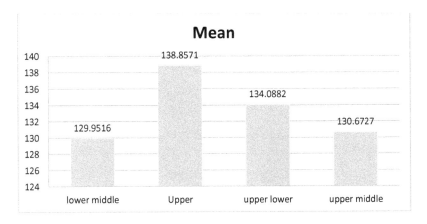

A careful inspection of Table 4.28 reveals that the calculated F value (1.133) is not significant at 0.05 level of significance (p>0.05). It means that there exist a no significant difference in the Personal values of urban boy adolescents of different socio-economic levels. It shows that socio-economic status does not affect the personal values of urban boy adolescents.

Therefor this may be that adolescents are more influenced by their peer group than by their parents. **Robert REL, Bengtson VL. (1999)** also found that in adolescence period, adolescents are more influenced by their peers then by parents. The families with low SES in urban areas also try their best to meet the educational needs of their children. And according to **Gupta (1992)** found that academic satisfaction was significantly related to their personality needs and personal values. Therefore there is no difference in the personal values of boy adolescents in urban areas of different SES.

g) **Effect of different dimensions of SES on personal values of girl adolescents from government school.**

TABLE-4.29

Mean, Standard Deviation & F Value of Personal Values of Adolescents with respect to Socio-Economic Status

Level of SES	Number of adolescents	Mean	Std. Deviation	Std. Error	F value	P value
Lower	2	114.5000	13.43503	9.50000	2.187	.072
lower middle	114	136.6404	14.10838	1.32137		
upper lower	71	139.1690	13.59830	1.61382		
upper middle	12	135.0000	9.97269	2.87887		

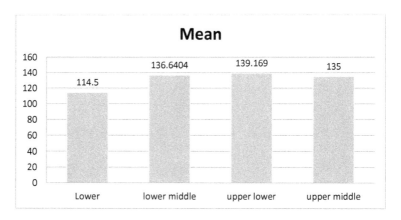

The perusal of table 4.29 reveals that the calculated F value (2.187) is not significant at 0.05 level of significance (p>0.05). It means that there exist a no significant difference in the Personal values of Government school girl adolescents of different socio-economic levels. It shows that socio-economic status does not affect the personal values of Government School girl adolescents.

It may be that the maximum girl adolescents studying in Government schools, as shown in the table, belong to lower middle and upper lower SES families in comparison to upper SES families. So due to low difference in their SES, there is no difference in their personal values.

h) **Effect of different dimensions of SES on personal values of boy adolescents from government school.**

TABLE-4.30

Mean, Standard Deviation & F Value of Personal Values of Adolescents with respect to Socio-Economic Status

Level of SES	Number of adolescents	Mean	Std. Deviation	Std. Error	F value	P value
Lower	8	119.3750	12.01116	4.24658		
lower middle	76	131.5526	19.38274	2.22335		
upper lower	103	135.0971	17.82624	1.75647	3.432	.010
upper middle	12	143.8333	9.27198	2.67659		

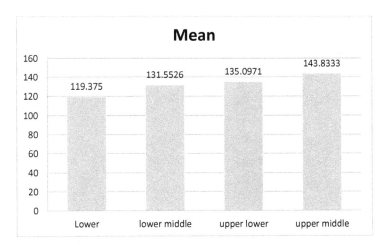

A glance at table 4.30 reveals that the calculated F value (3.432) is significant at 0.01 level of significance (p<0.01). It means that there exist a significant difference in the personal values of Government boy adolescents of different socio-economic levels. The above table reveals a significant difference between the mean scores of Lower, Upper lower, Lower Middle, Upper Middle & Upper class subjects. The result further reveals that those Government boy adolescents who belong to upper classes are having high personal values than the lower class Government school boy adolescents. Here we can say with 99% confidence that socio-economic status affect the Personal Values of boy adolescents studying in Government schools.

i) **Effect of different dimensions of SES on personal values of girls from non-government school.**

TABLE-4.31

Mean, Standard Deviation & F Value of Personal Values of Adolescents with respect to Socio-Economic Status

Level of SES	Number of adolescents	Mean	Std. Deviation	Std. Error	F value	P value
lower middle	57	127.0351	14.81428	1.96220		
Upper	34	135.4118	16.75694	2.87379		
upper lower	8	136.7500	7.88760	2.78869	3.015	.031
upper middle	101	129.2475	13.99100	1.39216		

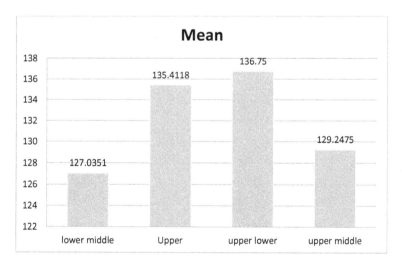

The perusal of table 4.31 reveals that the calculated F value (3.015) is significant at 0.05 level of significance (p<0.05). It means that there exist a significant difference in the personal values of Non-Government girl adolescents of different socio-economic levels. The above table reveals a significant difference between the mean scores of Lower, Upper lower, Lower Middle, Upper Middle & Upper class subjects. The result further reveals that those Non-Government girl adolescents who belong to upper classes are having high personal values than the lower class Non-Government girl adolescents. It shows that socio-economic status affect the Personal Values of Non-Government girl adolescents.

It may be because in Indian society girls spend most of their times within a family. They get values from their parents. **Magre, S. (2011)** found that there is significant difference in the religious, democratic, economic, knowledge, family prestige and health values of high SES and low SES students. Therefore girls of different SES have different personal values even though they studying in the same type of school.

j) **Effect of different dimensions of SES on personal values of boy adolescents from non- government school.**

TABLE-4.32

Mean, Standard Deviation & F Value of Personal Values of Adolescents with respect to Socio-Economic Status

Level of SES	Number of adolescents	Mean	Std. Deviation	Std. Error	F value	P value
lower middle	61	127.7377	17.83620	2.28369	.657	.579
Upper	26	132.3846	19.03277	3.73263		
upper lower	9	130.3333	15.70032	5.23344		
upper middle	104	127.7212	14.49570	1.42142		

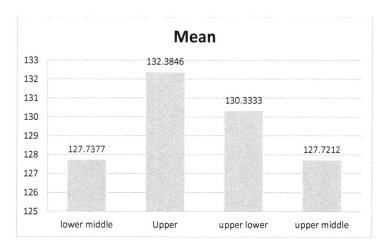

A glance at table 4.32 reveals that the calculated F value (.657) is not significant at 0.05 level of significance (p>0.05). It means that there exist a no significant difference in the Personal values of Non-Government School boy adolescents of different socio-economic levels. It shows that socio-economic status does not affect the personal values of Non-Government School boy adolescents.

This could be because due to studying in the same school environment, there is a no difference in the personal values of boy adolescents. This is in congruence with the study made by **Atul, M. et. al. (2015)** who revealed that there is no significant difference in the personal values of adolescents of different type of family.

k) **Effect of different dimensions of SES on personal values of adolescent.**

TABLE-4.33

Mean, Standard Deviation & F Value of Personal Values of l Adolescent with respect to Socio-Economic Status

Level of SES	Number of adolescents	Mean	Std. Deviation	Std. Error	F value	P value
Lower	10	118.4000	11.68285	3.69444	7.193	.000
lower middle	308	131.8442	16.83630	.95934		
Upper	62	134.9032	17.98425	2.28400		
upper lower	191	136.4555	16.02882	1.15980		
upper middle	229	129.6201	14.26841	.94288		

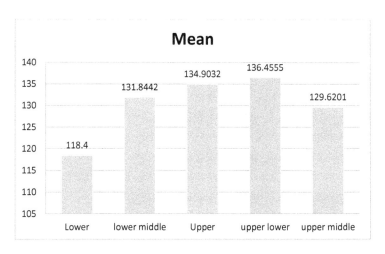

A glance at table 4.33 clearly reveals that the calculated F value (7.193) which is significant at 0.01 level of significance (p<0.01). It means that there exists a significant difference in the personal values of adolescents of different socio-economic levels. The above table reveals a significant difference between the mean scores of Lower, Upper lower, Lower Middle, Upper Middle & Upper class subjects. The result further reveals that those adolescents who belong to upper classes are having low personal values than the lower class adolescent. Here we can say with 99% of confidence that socio-economic status affect the Personal Values of adolescents. The result is in congruence with the studies made by

Hence in phase III, we observed that in most of the cases the result was found to be significantly different. Therefore the hypothesis III stating, **"There exists no significant difference between different dimensions of socio-economic status and personal values of adolescents"** is partially rejected.

PHASE IV- To see the relationship between self-confidence and mental health of adolescents.

a) **Relationship between self-confidence and mental health of girl and boy adolescents.**

TABLE- 4.34

Adolescents	N	r	Level of Significance
GA	400	-.532	0.01

| BA | 400 | -.606 | 0.01 |

GA=GIRL ADOLESCENTS, BA= BOYS ADOLESCENTS

A glance at table 4.34 reveals that relationship between SC and MH for GA (r = -0.532) as well as for BA (r = - 0.606), is significant at 0.01 level of significance. Magnitude of r indicates negative correlation which means that increase in self-confidence score leads to decrease in mental health scores and vice versa. In the present study, more self-confidence score means less self-confidence and less self-confidence score means more self-confidence thus we can conclude that with the increase in self-confidence of Girl and Boy adolescents there will be increase in their mental health and vice versa. So we can say with 99% confidence that SC and MH for GA and BA is positively significant regardless of gender.

Since self-confidence is not only a basic feature of mental health, but also a protective factor which is necessary for better mental health. On the other side low self-confidence may play a critical role in the development of mental disorder such as depression, anxiety, substance abuse etc. So gender plays no significant role.

b) Relationship between self- confidence and mental health of rural and urban girl adolescents.

TABLE-4.35

GA	N	r	Level of Significance
RGA	200	-.590	0.01
UGA	200	-.452	0.01

RGA= RURAL GIRL ADOLESCENT, UGA= URBAN GIRL ADOLESCENT

Table 4.35 presents the relationship between SC and MH of RGA (r = - 0.590) as well as UGA (r = - 0.452), is significant at 0.01 level of significance. Magnitude of r indicates negative correlation which means that increase in self-confidence scores leads to decrease in mental health scores and vice versa. In the present study, more self-confidence score means less self-confidence and less self- confidence score means more self-confidence thus we can conclude that with the increase in self-confidence of Rural Girl and Urban Girl adolescents there will be increase in their mental health and vice versa. So we are 99% confident that SC and MH of RGA as well as UGA is positively significant regardless of locality.

It is inferred from this that if the girl adolescents are mentally healthy they are highly self-self-confidence as well regardless of their locality, rural or urban, and vice versa. **Mehta et. al.** also concluded that highly assertive and self-self-confidence girls were found to be more adjusted (factor of mental health) in total as well as in social and emotional areas. Therefore in both the localities, rural as well as urban, mentally healthy girl adolescents are highly self-self-confidence.

c) **Relationship between self- confidence and mental health of rural and urban boy adolescents.**

TABLE-4.36

BA	N	r	Level of Significant
RBA	200	-.637	0.01
UBA	200	-.574	0.01

RBA= RURAL BOY ADOLESCENT, UBA= URBAN BOY ADOLESCENT

It is interesting to note from table 4.36 that relationship between SC and MH of UBA (r = -0.637) and RBA (r= -0.574), is significant at 0.01 level of significance. Magnitude of r indicates negative correlation which means that increase in self-confidence scores leads to decrease in mental health scores and vice versa. In the present study, more self-confidence score means less self-confidence and less self-confidence score means more self-confidence thus we can conclude that with the increase in self-confidence of Urban Boy and Rural Boys adolescents there will be increase in their mental health and vice versa. It means that there exists a positively significant relationship between SC and MH of boy adolescent regardless of locality.

A study of **Goel M. and Aggarwal P (2002)** is in congruence with the above result reporting that self-confident person feel himself to be socially fit, emotionally stable, intellectually adequate, successful, satisfied and self-reliant and having leadership qualities. Where emotional maturity and intelligence are the component of mental health. **Wankhade and Rokade (2011)** found that the average self-confidence of rural and urban, boys and girls are almost same. So if boy are self-confident them thy can be mentally healthy regardless of their locality.

d) **Relationship between self-confidence and mental health of rural government and Non- Government school girl adolescents.**

TABLE-4.37

GA	N	r	Level of Significant
RGSGA	100	-.701	0.01

| RNGSGA | 100 | -.501 | 0.01 |

RGSGA= RURAL GOVERNMENT SCHOOL GIRL ADOLESCENTS,
RNGSGA= RURAL NON- GOVERNMENT SCHOOL GIRL ADOLESCENTS

A perusal of table 4.37 reveals that the RGSGA (r = -0.701) as well as RNGSGA (r = -0.501), have a significant relationship at 0.01 level of significance between SC and MH. Magnitude of r indicates negative correlation which means that increase in self-confidence scores leads to decrease in mental health scores and vice versa. In the present study, more self-confidence score means less self-confidence and less self- confidence score means more self-confidence thus we can conclude that with the increase in self-confidence of Rural Government School and Rural Non-Government School Girls adolescents there will be increase in their mental health and vice versa.

It is inferred that there exists a positively significant relationship between SC and MH of rural girl adolescents regardless of type of school. **Tikkoo, Sangeeta (2006)** revealed that extroversion tendency enhance mental health whereas introversion tendency deteriorates mental health.

e) **Relationship between self-confidence and mental health of urban government and Non- Government school girl adolescents.**

TABLE-4.38

GA	N	r	Level of Significant
UGSGA	100	-.439	0.01
UNGSGA	100	-.530	0.01

UGSGA= URBAN GOVERNMENT SCHOOL GIRL ADOLESCENTS,
UNGSGA= URBAN NON- GOVERNMENT SCHOOL GIRL ADOLESCENTS

The value of 'r' depicted in table 4.38 for UGSGA (r= -0.439) and UNGSGA (r= -0.530), clearly shows that a significant relationship (at 0.01 level of significance) persists between SC and MH. Magnitude of r indicates negative correlation which means that increase in self-confidence scores leads to decrease in mental health scores and vice versa. In the present study, more self-confidence score means less self-confidence and less self- confidence score means more self-confidence thus we can conclude that with the increase in self-confidence of Urban Government School and Urban Non-Government School Girl adolescents there will be increase in their mental health and vice versa. It means that relationship between SC and MH of urban girl adolescent are positively significant regardless of type of school.

It can be inferred that in case of urban girl adolescents, whether they study in government school or in non-government school, if they are more self-self-confidence then they are mentally healthy as well. On the other hand, if they are not self-self-confidence they may be mentally unhealthy. Self-confidence guides the girl adolescents to be mentally healthy.

f) **Relationship between self- confidence and mental health of rural government and Non- Government school boy adolescents.**

TABLE-4.39

BA	N	r	Level of Significant
RGSBA	100	-.587	0.01
RNGSBA	100	-.551	0.01

RGSBA= RURAL GOVERNMENT SCHOOL BOY ADOLESCENTS,
RNGSBA= RURAL NON- GOVERNMENT SCHOOL BOY ADOLESCENTS

A perusal of table 4.39 reveals that the relationship between SC and MH of RGSBA (r = -0.587) and RNGSBA (r = -0.551), is significant at 0.01 level of significance. Magnitude of r indicates negative correlation which means that increase in self-confidence scores leads to decrease in mental health scores and vice versa. In the present study, more self-confidence score means less self-confidence and less self-confidence score means more self-confidence thus we can conclude that with the increase in self-confidence of Rural Government School and Rural Non-Government School Boys adolescents there will be increase in their mental health and vice versa. It means that there exists a positive significant relationship between SC and MH of rural boy adolescent regardless of type of school.

Reddy Sadananda, Prasad Kannekanti and Md. Hamza Ameer (2015) revealed that there is no any difference on self- esteem and stress of government and private school's students. It is believed that, a person possessing high level self-esteem will be self-confidence. That is why in both the schools, government as well as non-government, self-self-confidence boy adolescents are also mentally healthy.

g) **Relationship between self- confidence and mental health of urban government and Non- Government school boy adolescents.**

TABLE-4.40

BA	N	r	Level of Significant
UGSBA	100	-.736	0.01
UNGSBA	100	-.553	0.01

UGSBA= URBAN GOVERNMENT SCHOOL BOY ADOLESCENTS,
UNGSBA= URBAN NON- GOVERNMENT SCHOOL BOY ADOLESCENTS

A glance at table 4.40 reveals that the relationship between SC and MH of UGSGA (r = -0.736) and UNGSGA (r= -0.553), is significant at 0.01 level of significance. Magnitude of r indicates negative correlation which means that increase in self-confidence scores leads to decrease in mental health scores and vice versa. In the present study, more self-confidence score means less self-confidence and less self-confidence score means more self-confidence thus we can conclude that with the increase in self-confidence of Urban Government School and Urban Non-Government School Boys adolescents there will be increase in their mental health and vice versa. It is inferred from this that if the urban boy adolescents are self-self-confidence they are mentally healthy as well regardless they are studying in any type of school, government and non-government and vice versa.

h) **Relationship between self-confidence and mental health of total adolescents**

TABLE-4.41

Variables	N	R	Level of Significance
SC	800	-.570	0.01
MH			

SC= SELF-CONFIDENCE, MH= MENTAL HEALTH

The perusal of Table-4.41 indicates that the coefficient of correlation between Self-confidence and Mental Health of adolescents is -0.570 which is significant at 0.01 level of significance. Thus the null hypothesis i.e. "there is no significant relationship between self-confidence and Mental Health of adolescents", is rejected. Magnitude of r indicates negative correlation which means that increase in self-confidence scores leads to decrease in mental health scores and vice versa. In the present study, more self-confidence score means less self- confidence and less self- confidence score means more Self-confidence thus we can conclude that with the increase in self-confidence of adolescents there will be increase in their mental health and vice versa.

Self-confidence generate a kind of positive energy in us which gives positive outlook to our personality. Lack of self-confidence generates various mental health conditions in person such as depression, anxiety and stress due to which the mental health of the person is affected. **Selvaraj and Gnanadevan (2014)** revealed that there is a significant and negative correlation between self-confidence and different dimensions of stress like academic stress, interpersonal stress, intrapersonal stress, environmental stress and total stress.

In case of girl adolescent (GA) whether RGA and UGA, RGSGA or RNGSGA, UGSGA or UNGSGA there exists a positive and significant relationship between SC and MH. Similarly in case of boy adolescents (BA) (RBA or UBA, RGSBA or RNGSBA, UGSBA or UNGSBA) SC and MH are positively and significantly correlated with each other. On controlling gender, both boy and girl adolescent have a positive and significant relationship between SC and MH. It means that locality, type of school and gender does not play a significant role as for as this relationship between SC and MH is concerned.

Thus the above mentioned results clarifies that SC and MH of adolescents are positively and significantly correlated with each other. Therefore the IV hypothesis which predicted that, **"There exists no significant relationship between self-confidence and mental health of adolescents"**, is not confirmed and hence rejected.

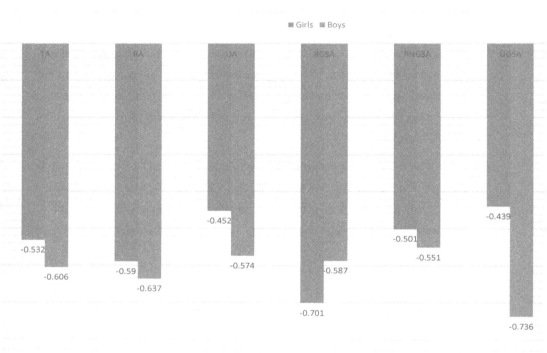

elationship between self-confidence and mental health of adolescents on the basis of locality gender a

PHASE V- To find the relationship between self- confidence and personal values of adolescents.

a) **Relationship between self- confidence and personal values of girl and boy adolescents.**

TABLE-4.42

Adolescents	N	r	Level of Significance
GA	400	-.600	0.01
BA	400	-.440	0.01

GA= GIRL ADOLESCENTS, BA= BOY ADOLESCENTS

A careful inspection of table 4.42 reveals that a significant relationship at 0.01 level of significance is found between SC and PV of GA (r = -0.600) and BA (r = -0.440). Magnitude of r indicates negative correlation which means that increase in self-confidence scores leads to decrease in Personal Values scores and vice versa. In the present study, more self-confidence score means less Self-confidence and less self-confidence score means more self-confidence thus we can conclude that with the increase in self-confidence of Girl and Boy adolescents there will be increase in their Personal Values and vice versa. It means that regardless of gender there exists a positively significant relationship between SC and PV of adolescents.

Following studies are consistent with the above result. **Mozhgan S. Mansoor et.al. (2012)** found that there is a significant and positive relationship between self-steam and hierarchy of values with social identity at male and female students. **Macnenen and Russel (2006)** believes that there is similarity between male and female values.

b) **Relationship between self- confidence and personal values of rural and urban girl adolescents.**

TABLE-4.43

GA	N	r	Level of Significance
RGA	200	-.466	0.01
UGA	200	-.372	0.01

RGA= RURAL GIRL ADOLESCENTS, UGA= URBAN GIRL ADOLESCENTS

Table 4.43 presents relationship between SC and PV of RGA (r = -0.466) and UGA (r = -0.372), which is significant at 0.01 level of significance. Magnitude of r indicates negative correlation which means that increase in self-confidence scores leads to decrease in Personal Values scores and vice versa. In the present study, more self-confidence score means less Self- confidence and less self- confidence score means more self-confidence thus we can conclude that with the increase in self-confidence of Rural Girl and Urban Girl adolescents there will be increase in their Personal Values and vice versa. The result reveals a positive and highly significant relationship between SC and PV of girl adolescents regardless of locality. According to **Branden (1994)** self-confidence in our ability to cope with the basic challenges of life and confidence our right to be successful and happy, the feeling being war the, achieve our values and energy.

c) **Relationship between self- confidence and personal values of rural and urban boy adolescents.**

TABLE-4.44

BA	N	r	Level of Significance
RBA	200	-.604	0.01
UBA	200	-.595	0.01

RBA= RURAL BOY ADOLESCENTS, UBA= URBAN BOY ADOLESCENTS

It is interesting to note from table 4.44 that relationship between SC and PV of UBA (r = -0.604) and RBA (r = -0.595), is significant at 0.01 level of significance. Magnitude of r indicates negative correlation which means that increase in self-confidence scores leads to decrease in Personal Values scores and vice versa. In the present study, more self-confidence score means less self-confidence and less self-confidence score means more self-confidence thus we can conclude that with the increase in self-confidence of Urban Boy and Rural Boy adolescents there will be increase in their Personal Values and vice versa. It means that there exists a positively significant relationship between SC and PV of boy adolescents regardless of locality.

Goel M. and Aggarwal P (2012) reported self Confidence is one of the personality trait which is a composite of a person's thoughts and feelings, strivings and hopes, fears and fantasies, his view of what he is, what he has been, what he might become, and his attitudes pertaining to his worth. On this basis we can say that self-confidence may enhance adolescent's personal values. So if boy adolescents are self-confidences they can have good personal values regardless of their locality.

d) **Relationship between self- confidence and personal values of rural government and Non- Government school girl adolescents.**

TABLE-4.45

GA	N	r	Level of Significance
RGSGA	100	-.578	0.01
RNGSGA	100	-.413	0.01

RGSGA= RURAL GOVERNMENT SCHOOL GIRL ADOLESCENTS, RNGSGA= RURAL NON-GOVERNMENT SCHOOL GIRL ADOLESCENTS

A glance at table 4.45 reveals that the relationship between SC and PV of RGSGA (r = -0.578) and RNGSGA (r= -0.413), is significant at 0.01 level of significance. Magnitude of r indicates negative correlation which means that increase in self-confidence scores leads to decrease in Personal Values scores and vice versa. In the present study, more self-confidence score means less self-confidence and less self-confidence score means more self-confidence thus we can conclude that with the increase in self-confidence of Rural Government School and Rural Non-Government School Girl adolescents there will be increase in their Personal Values and vice versa. It means that there exists a positively a significant relationship between SC and PV of rural girl adolescents regardless of type of school.

It can be inferred that in case of rural girl adolescents, whether they study in government school or in non-government school, if they are self-confidence then they have good personal values. On other hand, if they are not self-confidence then they may have poor values.

e) **Relationship between self- confidence and personal values of urban government and Non- Government school girl adolescents.**

TABLE-4.46

GA	N	r	Level of Significance
UGSGA	100	-.319	0.01
UNGSGA	100	-.532	0.01

UGSGA= URBAN GOVERNMENT SCHOOL GIRL ADOLESCENTS,
UNGSGA= URBAN NON-GOVERNMENT SCHOOL GIRL ADOLESCENTS

A careful inspection of table 4.46 reveals that the relationship between SC and PV of UGSGA (r = -0.319) and UNGSGA (r = -0.532), is significant at 0.01 level of significance. Magnitude of r indicates negative correlation which means that increase in self-confidence scores leads to decrease in Personal Values scores and vice versa. In the present study, more self-confidence score means less self-confidence and less self-confidence score means more self-confidence thus we can conclude that with the increase in self-confidence of Urban Government School and Urban Non-Government School Girl adolescents there will be increase in their Personal Values and vice versa. It means that there exists a positively significant relationship between SC and PV of urban girl adolescents regardless of type of school.

It is inferred that there exists a positively significantly relationship between SC and PV regardless of type of school. So we can say with 99% confidence that type of school has no significant role in the relationship between SC and PV of UGA. In urban society girls are taught of become self-confidence and to develop good values. They are taught to be modest and generous. So the girls mostly feel self-confidence whether they study in government or non-government school.

f) Relationship between self-confidence and personal values of rural government and Non-Government school boy adolescents.

TABLER- 4.47

BA	N	r	Level of Significance
RGSBA	100	-.635	0.01
RNGSBA	100	-.576	0.01

RGSBA= RURAL GOVERNMENT SCHOOL BOY ADOLESCENTS,
RNGSBA= RURAL NON-GOVERNMENT SCHOOL BOY ADOLESCENTS

A perusal of table 4.47 reveals that the relationship between SC and PV of RGSBA (r = -0.635) and RNGSBA (r = -0.576), is significant at 0.01 level of significance. Magnitude of r indicates negative correlation which means that increase in self-confidence scores leads to decrease in Personal Values scores and vice versa. In the present study, more self-confidence score means less self-confidence and less self-confidence score means more self-confidence thus we can conclude that with the increase in self-confidence of Rural Government School and Rural Non-Government

School Boy adolescents there will be increase in their Personal Values and vice versa. It means that there exists a positively significant relationship between SC and PV of rural boy adolescents regardless of type of school.

It inferred that as the level of self-confidence increases so does the level of personal values. On the other hand, low self-confidence signifies poor personal values. Therefore type of school does not play a significant role in this relationship between SC and PV.

g) **Relationship between self- confidence and personal values of urban government and Non- Government school boy adolescents.**

TABLE-4.48

BA	N	r	Level of Significance
UGSBA	100	-.710	0.01
UNGSBA	100	-.498	0.01

UGSBA= URBAN GOVERNMENT SCHOOL BOY ADOLESCENTS,
UNGSBA=URBAN NON-GOVERNMENT SCHOOL BOY ADOLESCENTS

A glance at table 4.48 reveals that the relationship between SC and PV of UGSGA (r = -0.710) and UNGSGA (r= -0.498), is significant at 0.01 level of significance. Magnitude of r indicates negative correlation which means that increase in self-confidence scores leads to decrease in Personal Values scores and vice versa. In the present study, more self-confidence score means less self-confidence and less self-confidence score means more self-confidence thus we can conclude that with the increase in self-confidence of Urban Government School and Urban Non-Government School Boy adolescents there will be increase in their Personal Values and vice versa. It means that there exists a positively significant relationship between SC and PV of urban boy adolescents regardless of type of school.

This might be due to the fact that irrespective of type of school in, urban areas parents tend to encourage boys more which may increase their self-confidence. That is why a positively significant relationship is observed between SC and PV of UGSBA as well as UNGSBA.

h) Relationship between self-confidence and personal values of total adolescents

TABLER-4.49

Variables	N	r	Level of Significance
SC	800	-.524	0.01
PV			

SC= SELF-CONFIDENCE, PV= PERSONAL VALUES

A glance a Table 4.49 reveals that adolescents relationship between self-confidence and personal value is (r = -0.524) significant at 0.01 level of significance Magnitude of r indicates negative correlation which means that increase in self-confidence scores leads to decrease in Personal Values scores and vice versa. In the present study, more self-confidence score means less Self-confidence and less self-confidence score means more Self-confidence thus we can conclude that with the increase in self-confidence of adolescents there will be increase in their Personal Values and vice versa. It means that there exists a positive and highly significant relationship between SC and PV of adolescents.

Personal values are important in helping to shape are lives. It can have a positive impact on one's self-confidences. When adolescents understand their personal values, it may provide them with a guideline for making positive choices and steering clear of negative situation. So if adolescents have high personal values then they may be self-confidence and vice versa.

It has been observed in case of relationship between SC and PV that locality, type of school or gender of adolescents plays no significant role. Therefore the above result and discussion clarifies that there exists a positively significant relationship between SC and PV of adolescents. Thus the V hypothesis predicting that **"There exists no significant relationship between self-confidence and personal values of adolescents"** is completely rejected.

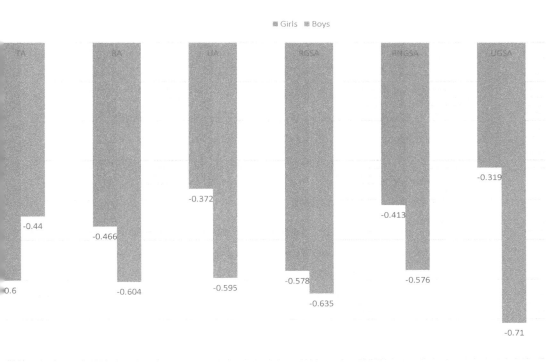

nship between self-confidence and personal values of adolescents on the basis of locality gender and

PHASE VI- To find the relationship between mental health and personal values of adolescents.

a) **Relationship between mental health and personal values of girls and boys adolescents.**

TABLE- 4.50

Adolescents	N	R	Level of Significance
GA	400	.636	0.01
BA	400	.751	0.01

GA= GIRL ADOLESCENTS, BA= BOY ADOLESCENTS

A careful inspection of table4.50reveals that a positive and significant relationship at 0.01 level of significant is found between MH and PV of GA (r = 0.636) and BA (r = 0.751). It means that there exists a positively significant relationship between MH and PV of Girls and Boys adolescents. It also means that high MH leads to high PV and vice versa in case of both GA as well as BA.

It could be because a mentally healthy person has the ability to make adjustment and has a sense of personal worth. He can give and accept love. A mentally healthy person forms his values keeping in mind the demand of the society. The findings are in congruence with that of **Andreas Maercker, Xiaochizhang et.al. (2015)** who indicate that personal values orientation are meaningful predictor of mental health and **Srividhya, V.; and Khadi, Pushpa, B. 2007** found that boys and girls did not differ in mental health status.

b) **Relationship between mental health and personal values of rural and urban girl adolescents.**

TABLE-4.51

GA	N	r	Level of Significance
RGA	200	.597	0.01
UGA	200	.663	0.01

RGA= RURAL GIRL ADOLESCENT, UGA= URBAN GIRL ADOLESCENT

Table 4.51presents a relationship between MH and PV of RGA (r=0.597) and UGA (r= 0.663). The result reveals a positive and highly significant relationship at 0.01

level of significance between MH and PV of girl adolescents regardless of locality. It means that there exists a positively significant relationship between MH and PV of Rural Girl and Rural Boy adolescents.

It is inferred from this that if the girl adolescents are mentally healthy they have good personal values as well regardless of their locality and vice versa. Mental health is the adolescent's adjustment with more effectiveness, satisfaction, happiness and socially acceptable behavior and the ability to face problems and accept the reality of life. It is an ability that can be achieved in rural as well as in urban surroundings. Adolescent girls belonging to rural areas can be mentally healthy just as those belonging to urban areas. **Singh, Arun kumar, Kumari Savita and Kumari Suprashna (2008)** also found that urban rural reason was not a significant determiner of mental health behavior. That is why in both the localities, rural as well as urban, mentally healthy girl adolescents have good personal values as well.

c) **Relationship between mental health and personal values of rural and urban boy adolescents.**

TALBE-4.52

BA	N	R	Level of Significance
RBA	200	.743	0.01
UBA	200	.758	0.01

RBA= RURAL BOY ADOLESCENT, UBA= URBAN BOY ADOLESCENT

It is interesting to note from table4.52 that relationship between MH and PV of RBA (r= 0.743) and UBA (r=0.758), is positively significant relationship at 0.01 level of significance. It means that there exists a positively significant relationship between MH and PV of Rural Girls and Rural Boys adolescents.

It can be inferred that RBA and UBA have good personal values because they are mentally healthy or vice versa. **A.K Menninger** states "mental health as the adjustment of human being to the world and to each other with a maximum of effectiveness and happiness." It is the ability to maintain an even temper, an intelligence, socially acceptable behavior and a happy behavior". On the other hand personal values are those characteristics and behavior that motivates us and guide our decisions. Personal values are the reflection of the highest principal of mind and thought. **Allport (1961)** define it as "A belief on which a man act by preference" so if the boy adolescents are mentally healthy they can have good personal values regardless of their locality.

d) **Relationship between mental health and personal values of rural government and Non- Government school girl adolescents.**

TABLE-4.53

GA	N	r	Level of Significance
RGSGA	100	.613	0.01
RNGSGA	100	.569	0.01

RGSGA= RURAL GOVERNMENT SCHOOL GIRL ADOLESCENTS,
RNGSGA= RURAL NON-GOVERNMENT SCHOOL GIRL ADOLESCENTS

A glance at table 4.53 reveals that the relationship between MH and PV of RGSGA (r=0.613) and RNGSGA (r=0.569), is positively and highly significant at 0.01 level of significance. It means that there exists a positively significant relationship between MH and PV of Rural Government School Girl and Rural Non-Government School Girl adolescents.

So it means that type of school has no significant role in the relationship between MH and PV of rural girl adolescents. **Bindo (2016)** also found that the students from government and private schools have similar emotional stability (Component of mental health).

e) **Relationship between mental health and personal values of urban government and Non- Government school girl adolescents.**

TABLER- 4.54

GA	N	r	Level of Significance
UGSGA	100	.633	0.01
UNGSGA	100	.631	0.01

UGSGA= URBAN GOVERNMENT SCHOOL GIRL ADOLESCENTS,
UNGSGA= URBAN NON-GOVERNMENT SCHOOL GIRL ADOLESCENTS

A perusal of table 4.54 reveals that the UGSGA (r = 0.633) and UNGSGA (r=0.631), have a positive and highly significant relationship at 0.01 level of significance between MH and PV. It means that there exists a positively significant relationship between MH and PV of Urban Government School Girl and Urban Non-Government School Girl adolescents.

It could be because girls are empathetic, submissive, patient and have stability in their emotions. So they are mentally healthy as well as have good personal values, whether they study in government schools or in non-government schools.

f) **Relationship between mental health and personal values of rural government and Non- Government school boy adolescents.**

TABLE- 4.55

BA	N	r	Level of Significance
RGSBA	100	.773	0.01
RNGSBA	100	.697	0.01

RGSBA= RURAL GOVERNMENT SCHOOL BOY ADOLESCENTS,
RNGSBA= RURAL NON-GOVERNMENT SCHOOL BOY ADOLESCENTS

From the content of the table 4.55 it is revealed that RGSBA(r=0.773) and RNGSBA (r=0.697), have a positive and highly significant relationship at 0.01 level of significance between MH and PV. It means that there exists a positively significant relationship between MH and PV of Rural Government School Boy and Rural Non-Government School Boy adolescents.

Long and shiffam (2000) states that "Personal values are relevant to all areas of life as they influence one's preferred choice of behaviour in any given situation and are able to "guide actions, attitudes, judgments, and comparisons across specific objects and situations". It reflect one's ability to deal with their environment. So if boy adolescents are mentally healthy they have good personal values also regardless of whether they study in government or in non-government school.

g) **Relationship between different mental health and personal values of urban government and Non- Government school boy adolescents.**

TABLE-4.56

BA	N	r	Level of Significance
UGSBA	100	.766	0.01
UNGSBA	100	.748	0.01

UGSBA= URBAN GOVERNMENT SCHOOL BOY ADOLESCENTS,
UNGSBA= URBAN NON-GOVERNMENT SCHOOL BOY ADOLESCENTS

It is interesting to note from table 4.56 that relationship between MH and PV of UGSGA (r= 0.766) and UNGSGA (r=0.748), is positively significant relationship at 0.01 level of significance. It means that there exists a positively significant relationship between MH and PV of Urban Government School Boy and Urban Non-Government School Boy adolescents.

It is because boys are emotionally stable. The emotional stability may be cited as Calmness of mind and it is free from anxiety and depression (**Hay and Ashman 2003**). Emotional stability is a factor of mental health. An emotionally stable person also have good mental health. **Kaur (2013)** also revealed that there was not any significant difference in various areas of emotional stability of government and private school. And a mentally healthy person shows a healthy values and self-concept. So type of school does not play a significant role in the relationship between MH and PV.

h) **Relationship between mental health and personal values of total adolescents**

TABLE- 4.57

Variables	N	r	Level of Significance
MH	800	.703	0.01
PV			

MH= MENTAL HEALTH, PV= PERSONAL VALUE

A glance at Table 4.57 reveals that the adolescent relationship between MH and PV is positive (r = .703) as well as highly significant at 0.01 level of significance. It means that there exists a positive and highly significant relationship between Mental Health and Personal Values Adolescents.

It is inferred that adolescent's mental health is related to their personal values. A mentally healthy person shows a homogeneous organization of desirable attitudes, healthy values and righteous self-concept and a scientific perception of the world as a whole. Several psychologists like **Erikson (1936), Rogers (1969), Hurlock (1972)** have expressed their views in a similar tone.

It has been observed in case of relationship between mental health and personal values that locality, type of school or gender of adolescents plays no significant role. Therefore the above result and discussion clarifies with 99% confidence that there exists a positively significant relationship between mental health and personal values of adolescents. Thus the VI hypothesis predicting that **"There is no significant difference between mental health and personal values of adolescents"** is completely rejected.

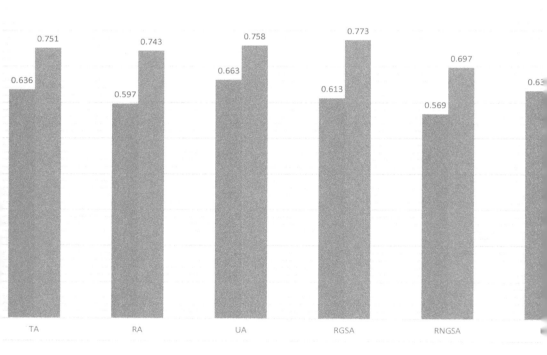

ionship between mental health and personal values of adolescents on the basis of locality, g
school

PHASE VII (A)-To find out the effect of locality on the self-confidence of adolescents.

a) **Comparison between rural and urban girl adolescents.**

TABLE- 4.58

Significance of difference between RGA & UGA on SC

Variables	RGA		UGA		t	P
	M	SD	M	SD		
SC	24.1900	9.74158	27.5750	9.30037	-3.554	0.00

SC= Self-Confidence, RGA= Rural Girl Adolescents & UGA= Urban Girl Adolescents

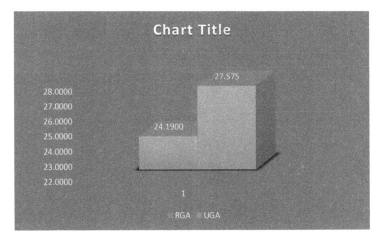

Effect of Locality on Self- Confidence of Girl Adolescents

A careful inspection of table 4.58 reveals that the calculated t value (-3.554) is significant at 0.01 level of significance (p<0.01). It means that a significant difference is found between the self-confidence of RGA and UGA.

It also means that locality has a significant effect on SC of Girl adolescent. The mean score of UGA is 27.5750 and RGA is 24.1900. The mean score of UGA is greater than the mean score of RGA, but according to manual of the test lower the score, higher would be self-confidence so the result indicate that RGA are more confident than UGA.

It could be because girls spend most of their time with their family. In urban areas, most of parents are working, so they do not give much time to their children. And when parental involvement is limited, children typically receive low encouragement.

They have no one reflecting back to them that they are worthwhile, admirable or interesting which may decrease their self-confidence. Whereas in rural areas family still spend quality time together. They develop the feeling of trust in them and this belief may built self-confidence in them. The result is in congruence with that of **Fareen Fatima (2015)** who found that the self-confidence of adolescents from rural area is higher is in comparison to adolescents from urban areas.

b) **Comparison between rural and urban boy adolescents.**

TABLE- 4.59

Significance of difference between RBA & UBA on SC

Variables	RBA		UBA		T	P
	M	SD	M	SD		
SC	25.6750	10.13424	25.2650	10.21354	.403	.687

SC= Self- Confidence, RBA= Rural Boy Adolescents & UBA= Urban Boy Adolescents

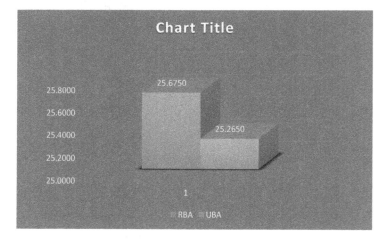

Effect of Locality on Self- Confidence of Boy Adolescents

A glance at table 4.59 reveals that the calculated t value (.403) is not significant at 0.05 level of significance (p>0.05). It means that there exist no significant difference between RBA and UBA on SC.

It show that locality has no effect on the SC of Boy Adolescents. This may be because boys in both urban and rural areas get equal support from the family. According to **Rehman Abzaizul, Mohmood Rehman Abdull et.al. (2018)** there is a significant relationship between parental support and adolescent self-concept. They also found that there is a significant relationship between parental support and adolescent self- esteem.

Therefore no difference has been found in the self-confidence of rural and urban boy adolescents.

c) **Comparison between rural government and urban government girl adolescents.**

TABLE- 4.60

Significance of difference between RGSGA & UGSGA on SC

Variables	RGSGA		UGSGA		t	P
	M	SD	M	SD		
SC	26.3100	10.37742	28.0800	9.61237	-1.251	.212

SC= Self- Confidence, RGSGA= Rural Government School Girl Adolescents & UGSGA= Urban Government School Girl Adolescents

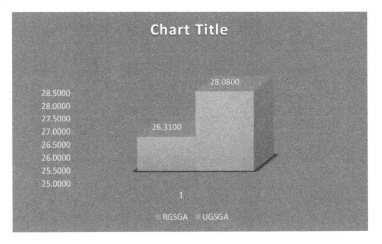

Effect of Locality on Self- Confidence of Government School Girl Adolescents

A perusal of table 4.66 reveals that the calculated t value (-1.251) is not significant at 0.05 level of significance (p>0.05). It means that there exist no significant difference between RGSGA and UGSGA on SC.

It is inferred from the above mentioned result that locality does not affect the self-confidence of government school girl adolescents. The reason for this may be that the environment of rural and urban government schools is similar and also SES of students studying in them is also almost the same. Therefore no difference has been found in the self-confidence of girls studying in government schools in urban as well as in rural areas due to similar family and school environment.

d) **Comparison between rural government and urban government boy adolescents.**

TABLE-4.61

Significance of difference between RGSBA & UGSBA on SC

Variables	RGSBA		UGSBA		T	P
	M	SD	M	SD		
SC	25.0500	10.71521	26.8000	10.39522	-1.172	.243

SC= Self- Confidence, RGSBA= Rural Government School Boy Adolescents
UGSBA= Urban Government School Boy Adolescents

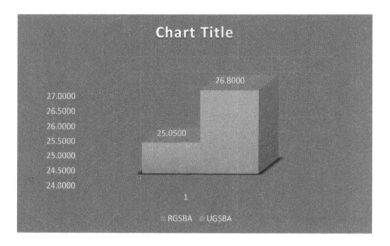

Effect of Locality on Self- Confidence of Government School Boy Adolescents

A study of table 4.61 reveals that the calculated value of t (1.172) is not significant at 0.05 level of significance (p>0.05). It means that there exist no significant difference between RGSBA and UGSBA on SC.

It is inferred that both RGSBA and UGSBA have equal level of self-confidence. The schools are poor or rich with respect to the environment they provide for their students. And the environment of government schools regardless of locality is almost the same. **Dr. Jyoti (2015)** also found that area does not play a significant role in high or low level of self-confidence of adolescents. Therefore there is no significant difference between the self-confidence of rural and urban government school boy adolescents.

e) **Comparison between rural non- government and urban non-government girl adolescents.**

TABLE-4.62

Significance of difference between RNGSGA & UNGSGA on SC

Variables	RNGSGA		UNGSGA		t	P
	M	SD	M	SD		
SC	22.0700	8.60145	27.0700	8.99748	-4.017	.000

SC= Self- Confidence, RNGSGA= Rural Non-Government School Girl Adolescents & UNGSGA= Urban Non-Government School Girl Adolescents

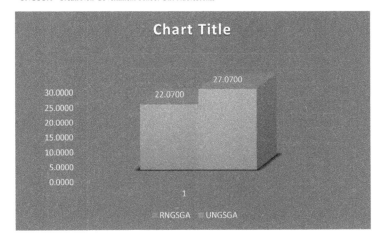

Effect of Locality on Self- Confidence of Non-Government School Girl Adolescents

From the content of table 4.62 it is revealed that the calculated t value (-4.017) is significant at 0.01 level of significance (p<0.01). It means that a significant difference is found between the self-confidence of RNGSGA and UNGSGA. The mean score of RNGSGA is 22.0700 and UNGSGA is 27.0700. The mean score of UNGSGA is greater than the mean score of RNGSGA, but according to manual of the test lower the score, higher would be self-confidence so the result indicate that RNGSGA is more confident than UNGSGA.

The reason for this may be that there is a huge difference in the environment of non-government schools in rural and urban areas. Students studying in non-government schools in urban areas face study pressure and competition which can create stress in them. And stress affect the self-confidence of the child. **Selvaraj and Gnanadevan (2014)** reveals that there is a significant and negative relationship between self-confidence and different dimensions of stress such as academic stress, environmental stress and total stress. And **William M.W (2010)** reveals that female students display more psychological stress and depression symptoms. Here the self-confidence of RNGSGA is greater that the UNGSGA may be because rural girl adolescents face less psychological stress and depression symptoms.

f) **Comparison between rural non- government and urban non-government boy adolescents.**

TABLE-4.63

Significance of difference between RNGSBA & UNGSBA on SC

Variables	RNGSBA		UNGSBA		t	P
	M	SD	M	SD		
SC	26.3000	9.53092	23.7300	9.84204	1.876	.062

SC= Self- Confidence, RNGSBA= Rural Non-Government School Boy Adolescents & UNGSBA= Urban Non- School Boy Adolescents

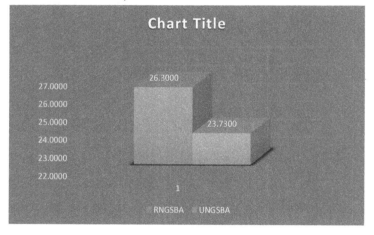

Effect of Locality on Self- Confidence of Non-Government School Boy Adolescents

A glance at table 4.63 reveals that the calculated t value is 1.876 which is not significant at 0.05level of significance (p>0.05).It means that there exist no significant difference between RNGSBA and UNGSBA on SC.

The reason for this may be that even though there is a difference in the environment of non-government schools in urban and rural areas and students studying in non- government school in urban areas have higher academic stress. But because boys have lower stress level then girls. Therefore there is no difference between the self-confidence of rural and urban non-government school boy adolescents. **Legy**

(2018) also found that women are more likely to be diagnostic with anxiety disorders as compare to men.

g) **Comparison between rural and urban government school adolescents.**

TABLE- 4.64

Significance of difference between RGSA & UGSA on SC

Variables	RGSA		UGSA		t	P
	M	SD	M	SD		
SC	25.6800	10.54007	27.4400	10.00685	-1.713	.088

SC= Self- Confidence, RGSA= Rural Government School Adolescents &
UGSA= Urban Government School Adolescents

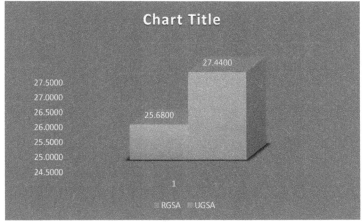

Effect of Locality on Self- Confidence of Government School Adolescents

A careful inspection of table 4.64 reveals that the calculated t value (-1.713) is not significant at 0.05 level of significance (p>0.05). It means that there exist no significant difference between RGSA and UGSA on SC.

It show that locality has no effect on the SC of Government School Adolescents. The reason for this may be that there is no difference in the self-confidence of RGSA and UGSA due to studying in similar school environment.

h) **Comparison between rural and urban non-government adolescents.**

TABLE- 4.65

Significance of difference between RNGSA & UNGSA on SC

Variables	RNGSA		UNGSA		t	P
	M	SD	M	SD		
SC	24.1850	9.30017	25.4000	9.55334	-1.289	.198

SC= Self- Confidence, RNGSA= Rural Non-Government School Adolescents &
UNGSA= Urban Non-Government School Adolescents

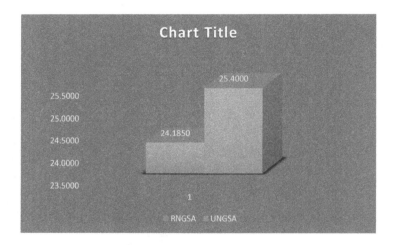

Effect of Locality on Self- Confidence of Non-Government School Adolescents

A perusal of table 4.65 reveals that the calculated t value (-1.289) is not significant at 0.05 level of significance (p>0.05). It means that there exist no significant difference between RNGSA and UNGSA on SC.

It show that locality has no effect on the SC of Non-Government School Adolescents.

i) **Comparison between rural and urban adolescents.**

TABLE- 4.66

Significance of difference between RA & UA on SC

Variables	RA		UA		T	P
	M	SD	M	SD		
SC	24.9325	9.95518	26.4200	9.82369	-1.127	0.182

SC= Self- Confidence, RA= Rural Adolescents & UA= Urban Adolescents

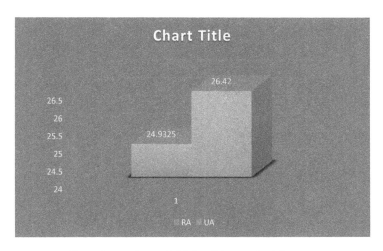

Effect of Locality on Self-Confidence of adolescents.

A perusal of table 4.66 reveals that the calculated t value (-1.127) is not significant at 0.05 level of significance (p>0.05). It means that there exist no significant difference between RA and UA on SC.

It is inferred that locality does not affect the self-confidence of adolescents. Adolescents of rural as well as urban areas are equally self-confident. The above result is in congruence with that of **Dr. Jyoti (2015)** who found that area does not play a significant role in high or low level of self-confidence of adolescents.

PHASE VII (B)-To find out the effect of locality on the Mental Health of adolescents.

a) **Comparison between rural and urban girl adolescents.**

TABLE- 4.67

Significance of difference between RGA & UGA on MH

Variables	RGA		UGA		t	P
	M	SD	M	SD		
MH	77.1700	9.08094	74.8400	9.13299	2.558	0.011

MH- Mental Health, RGA= Rural Girl Adolescents & UGA= Urban Girl Adolescents

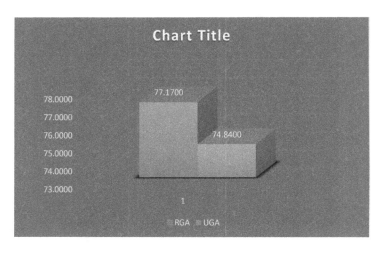

Effect of Locality on Mental Health of Girl adolescents.

A perusal of table 4.67 reveals that the calculated t value (2.558) is significant at 0.05 level of significance (p<0.05). It means that there a significant difference between RGA and UGA on MH. The mean score of RGA is 77.1700 and UGA is 74.8400. The mean score of RGA is greater than the mean score of UGA, so the result indicate that the mental health of RGA is more than UGA.

It shows that locality affects the MH of girl adolescents. The reason for this may be that the environment of the urban area is more tense than that of the rural area. Everyone wants to maintain their status in the society. The brightness of the urban area gives rise to many desires in them. And if their wishes are not fulfilled, they become stressed. In contrast, the people of rural areas lead a simple life. That is why the mental health of girls in rural area is found to be higher than that of girls in urban area.

b) **Comparison between rural and urban boy adolescents.**

TABLE- 4.68

Significance of difference between RBA & UBA on MH

Variables	RBA		UBA		t	P
	M	SD	M	SD		
MH	74.6050	10.47222	75.4300	10.79294	-.776	.438

MH- Mental Health, RBA= Rural Boy Adolescents & UBA= Urban Boy Adolescents

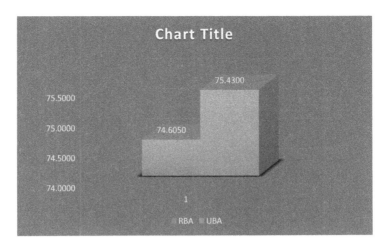

Effect of Locality on Mental Health of Boy Adolescents

A perusal of Table 4.68 reveals that the calculated t value (-.776) is not significant at 0.05 level of significance (p>0.05). It means that there exists no significant difference between RBA and UBA on MH.

It is inferred that locality does not effect on the MH of Boy Adolescents. It may be that boy adolescent of rural as well as urban areas are equally adjusted and adjustment level affect the mental health because **Srividhya, V.; and Khadi, Pushpa, B (2007)** reveals that mental health significantly correlated to adjustment problems, indicating higher the problem lower the mental health.

c) **Comparison between rural government and urban government girl adolescents.**

TABLE- 4.69

Significance of difference between RGSGA & UGSGA on MH

Variables	RGSGA M	RGSGA SD	UGSGA M	UGSGA SD	t	P
MH	77.8600	10.21785	77.2200	8.44899	.483	.630

MH= Mental Health, RGSGA= Rural Government School Girl Adolescents & UGSGA= Urban Government School Girl Adolescents

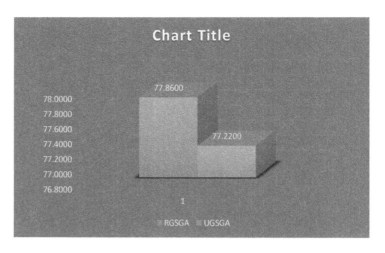

Effect of Locality on Mental Health of Government School Girl Adolescents

A glance at table 4.69 reveals that the calculated t value (.483) is not significant at 0.05 level of significance (p>0.05). It means that there exist no significant difference between RGSGA and UGSGA on MH.

It is inferred that locality does not affect the MH of Government School Girl Adolescents. Girl adolescents spend most of their time at home or in school. The school environment plays a significant role in the development of adolescents. It is quite evident that the school environment can help students develop qualities of adjustment and self-confidence. Which impact the mental health of adolescents because **Srividhya, V.; and Khadi, Pushpa, B (2007)** reveals that mental health significantly correlated to adjustment problems, indicating higher the problem lower the mental health and **Tikkoo, Sangeeta (2006)** revealed that extroversion tendency enhance mental health whereas introversion tendency deteriorates mental health. But rural areas in this study are very close to urban areas or rather they are peri-urban. Therefore there is not much difference in the environment of government schools in rural and urban areas. That is why no difference has been found in the mental health of girl adolescents of government school of rural and urban areas.

d) **Comparison between rural government and urban government boy adolescents.**

TABLE-4.70

Significance of difference between RGSBA & UGSBA on MH

Variables	RGSBA		UGSBA		t	P
	M	SD	M	SD		
MH	76.0600	11.19598	75.9400	11.48457	.075	.940

MH= Mental Health, RGSBA= Rural Government School Boy Adolescents &UGSBA= Urban Government School Boy Adolescents

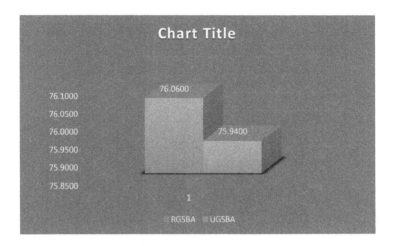

Effect of Locality on Mental Health of Government School Boy Adolescents

A perusal of table 4.70 reveals that the calculated t value (0.75) is not significant at 0.05 level of significance (p>0.05). It means that there exist no significant difference between RGSBA and UGSBA on MH.

It shows that locality does not affect the MH of Government School Boy Adolescents. In the above result we have found that there is no difference in the mental health of government school girl adolescents of rural and urban areas. The result is in congruence with the findings **Singh, Arun Kumar, Kumari Savita and Kumari Suprashna (2008)** has found that there is a negative impact of lower SES on development of mental health behavior. However, there is no impact of urban rural region on mental health behavior. **Mittal A. (2008)** found that the mental health of secondary level students of rural as well as urban localities are same.

Similarly **Sarita, Dahiya, Rajani and Pushpanjali (2015)** found that the mental health of boys and girls of government senior secondary school are same.

Therefore no difference has found in the mental health of government school boy adolescents of rural and urban areas.

e) **Comparison between rural non- government and urban non-government girl adolescents.**

TABLE-4.71

Significance of difference between RNGSGA & UNGSGA on MH

Variables	RNGSGA		UNGSGA		t	P
	M	SD	M	SD		
MH	76.4800	7.77133	72.4600	9.21069	3.336	.001

MH= Mental Health, RNGSGA= Rural Non-Government School Girl Adolescents &
UNGSGA= Urban Non-Government School Girl Adolescents

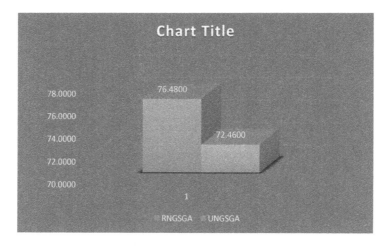

Effect of Locality on Mental Health of Non-Government School Girl Adolescents

A glance at Table 4.71 reveals that the calculated t value (3.336) is significant at 0.05 level of significance (p<0.05). It means that a significant difference is found between the MH of RNGSGA and UNGSGA. The mean score of RNGSGA is 76.4800 and UNGSGA is 72.4600. The mean score of RNGSGA is greater than the mean score of UNGSGA, so the result indicate that the mental health of RNGSGA is more than UNGSGA.

The school environment plays a significant role in the development of adolescents. Non-Government schools take the responsibility and special care in the all-round development of the adolescents. It may be that there is a lot of difference in the non-government school environment in rural and urban areas. Students studying in non-government schools in urban areas have a large burden of extra activities. There is competition to get good marks in all activities. There is a fear of being dropped from school if the marks are not good. Which boosts their anxiety and affect their mental health **RadhikaKapur (2020)** reported when anxiety takes place in a major form, it has deter mental effects upon health and well-being of the individuals. **Legy, 2018** also found that women are more likely to be diagnostic with anxiety disorders as compared to men.

Whereas in non-government school in rural areas no such pressure is put on the students. Due to which their mental health may be good. Therefore the mental health of girl adolescents of non-government schools in rural areas is higher than girls in urban areas.

f) **Comparison between rural non- government and urban non-government boy adolescents.**

TABLE-4.72

Significance of difference between RNGSBA & UNGSBA on MH

Variables	RNGSBA		UNGSBA		t	P
	M	SD	M	SD		
MH	73.1500	9.52972	74.9200	10.08617	-1.276	.204

MH= Mental Health, RNGSBA= Rural Non-Government School Boy Adolescents & UNGSBA= Urban Non- School Boy Adolescents

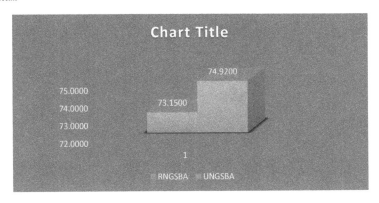

Effect of Locality on Mental Health of Non-Government School Boy Adolescents

A careful inspection of table 4.72 clearly reveals that calculated t value (-1.276) is not significant at 0.05 level of significance (p>0.05). It means that there exist no significant difference between RNGSBA and UNGSBA on MH.

It show that locality does not affect the MH of Non-Government School Boy Adolescents. As we discussed in table 4.78 that students studying in non-government school in urban areas have great concern to succeed in life. They are forced to score good marks. But the probable reason for the above result could be that boys are less affected by all these things than girls.

Therefore there is no significant difference in mental health of boys studying in non-government school in rural and urban areas.

g) **Comparison between rural and urban government school adolescents.**

TABLE- 4.73

Significance of difference between RGSA & UGSA on MH

Variables	RGSA		UGSA		t	P
	M	SD	M	SD		
MH	76.9600	10.72912	76.5800	10.07677	.365	.715

MH= Mental Health, RGSA= Rural Government School Adolescents & UGSA= Urban Government School Adolescents

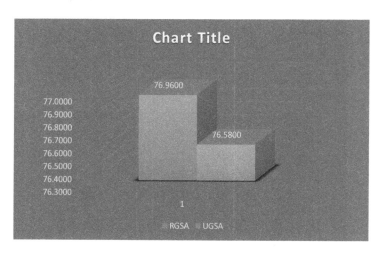

Effect of Locality on Mental Health of Government School Adolescents

A glance at table 4.73 clearly reveals that the calculated t value (.365) is not significant at 0.05 level of significance (p>0.05). It means that there exist no significant difference between RGSA and UGSA on MH.

It shows that locality does not affect the MH of Government School Adolescents. In table 4.70 we found that there is no difference in mental health of girls from government school in urban and rural areas and from table 4.71 we found that there is also no difference in mental health of boys from government school in urban and rural areas. **Srividhya, V.; and Khadi, Pushpa, B (2007)** also found that the mental health of boy and girl adolescents are same. Similarly **Sarita, Dahiya, Rajani and Pushpanjali (2015)** also found that there is no significance difference in mental health of boys and girls of government senior secondary school.

Therefore in total way we can say that there is no difference in the mental health of adolescents of government schools in urban and rural areas.

h) **Comparison between rural and urban non-government adolescents.**

TABLE- 4.74

Significance of difference between RNGSA & UNGSA on MH

Variables	RNGSA		UNGSA		t	P
	M	SD	M	SD		
MH	74.8150	8.83237	73.6900	9.71265	1.212	.226

MH= Mental Health, RNGSA= Rural Non-Government School Adolescents & UNGSA= Urban Non-Government School Adolescents

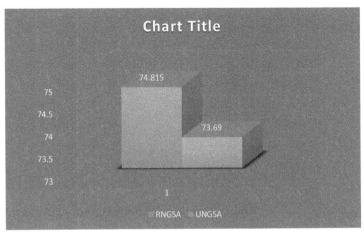

Effect of Locality on Mental Health of Non-Government School Adolescents

A perusal of Table 4.74 reveals that the calculated t value (1.212) is not significant at 0.05 level of significance (p>0.05). It means that there exist no significant difference between RNGSA and UNGSA on MH.

It shows that locality does not effect on the MH of Non-Government School Adolescents. A study by **Singh, Arun Kumar, Kumari Savita and Kumari Suprashna (2008)** is in congruence with the above result reporting that urban, rural region is not a determiner of mental health behavior. **Sarita, Dahiya, Rajani and Pushpanjali (2015)** also found that the mental health of boys and girls of private senior secondary school are same.

i) **Comparison between rural and urban adolescents.**

TABLE- 4.75

Significance of difference between RA & UA on MH

Variables	RA		UA		t	P
	M	SD	M	SD		
MH	75.8875	9.87287	75.1350	9.98931	1.072	0.284

MH- Mental Health, RA= Rural Adolescents & UA= Urban Adolescents

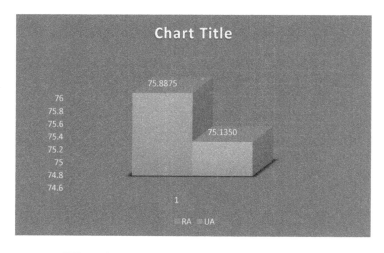

Effect of Locality on Mental Health of adolescents.

A glance at table 4.75 clearly reveals that the calculated t value (1.072) is not significant at 0.05 level of significance (p>0.05). It means that there exists no significant difference between the mental health of RA and UA.

It is inferred that locality does not affect the MH of Adolescents. The result is in congruence with that of **Singh, Arun Kumar, Kumari Savita and Kumari Suprashna (2008)** who found that urban and rural region is not a determiner of mental health behavior.

PHASE VII (C)- To find out the effect of locality on the Personal Values of adolescents.

a) **Comparison between rural and urban girl adolescents.**

TABLE- 4.76

Significance of difference between RGA & UGA on PV

Variables	RGA		UGA		t	P
	M	SD	M	SD		
PV	136.2450	15.07152	131.0200	14.05122	3.586	0.00

PV- Personal Values, RGA= Rural Girl Adolescents & UGA= Urban Girl Adolescents

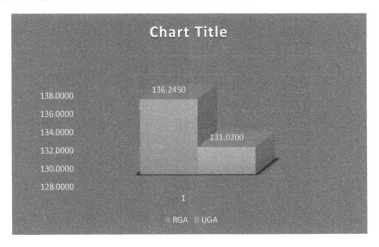

Effect of Locality on Personal Values of Girl adolescents.

A glance a table 4.76 reveals that the calculated t value (3.586) is significant at 0.05 level of significance (p<0.05). It means that a significant difference is found between the Personal Values of RGA and UGA.

It shows that Locality has effect on PV of UGA and RGA. The mean score of RGA is 136.2450 and UGA is 131.0200. The mean score of RGA is greater than the mean score of UGA, so the result indicate that RGA has more personal values than UGA. It may be that Indian society believes in developing more personal values among girls than among boys and these expectations are higher in rural areas, whereas in urban areas both girls and boys are treated equally. It may also be that due to very busy schedule in urban areas parents are unable to pay attention to the development of personal values in their children. Therefore the personal values of girl adolescents in rural areas are higher than the girls in urban areas.

b) **Comparison between rural and urban boy adolescents.**

TABLE- 4.77

Significance of difference between RBA & UBA on PV

Variables	RBA		UBA		t	P
	M	SD	M	SD		
PVS	130.0150	17.57925	132.2300	17.37806	-1.267	.206

PV- Personal Values, RBA= Rural Boy Adolescents & UBA= Urban Boy Adolescents

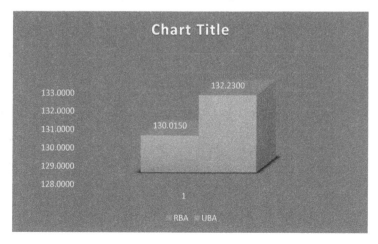

Effect of Locality on Personal Values of Boy Adolescents

A glance at table 4.77 reveals that the calculated t value (-1.267) which is not significant at 0.05 level of significance (p>0.05). It means that there exist no significant difference between RBA and UBA on PV.

It is inferred that locality does not affect the PV of Boy Adolescents. It may be that the child also develops personal values from the home environment. Family members develop values in the children. **Benjamin, B. Maxwell (2011)** found that the moral, personal, academic, social and aesthetic values of students are similar irrespective to the level of home environment (High, moderate and low). This means the home environment has no effect on personal values. Families of different SES level lives in both rural and urban areas of Dehradun district. Therefore no difference has been found in the personal values of boy adolescents living in rural and urban areas.

c) **Comparison between rural government and urban government girl adolescents.**

TABLE- 4.78

Significance of difference between RGSGA & UGSGA on PV

Variables	RGSGA		UGSGA		t	P
	M	SD	M	SD		
PVS	138.0200	15.90564	136.5800	11.55066	.733	.465

PV= Personal Values, RGSGA= Rural Government School Girl Adolescents & UGSGA= Urban Government School Girl Adolescents

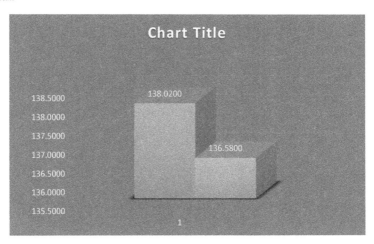

Effect of Locality on Personal Values of Government School Girl Adolescents

A careful inspection of table 4.78 clarifies that the calculated t value (.733) is not significant at 0.05 level of significance (p>0.05). It means that there exist no significant difference between RGSGA and UGSGA on PV.

It shows that locality does not affect the PV of Government School Girl Adolescents. It may be that there is no significant difference in the environment of government schools in rural and urban areas and girls are more affected by their family environment as they spend more and more time with their family members. And the home environment has no effect on the child's personal values **Benjamin, B. Maxwell (2011).** Therefore there is no difference in the personal values of girls from government school in urban and rural areas.

d) **Comparison between rural government and urban government boy adolescents.**

TABLE-4.79

Significance of difference between RGSBA & UGSBA on PV

Variables	RGSBA		UGSBA		t	P
	M	SD	M	SD		
PVS	133.9600	17.50089	133.6300	19.23310	.127	.899

PV= Personal Values, RGSBA= Rural Government School Boy Adolescents &UGSBA= Urban Government School Boy Adolescents

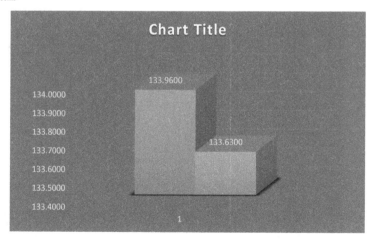

Effect of Locality on Personal Values of Government School Boy Adolescents

A perusal of Table 4.79 reveals that the calculated t value (.127) is not significant at 0.05 level of significance (p>0.05). It means that there exist no significant difference between RGSBA and UGSBA on PV.

It is inferred that locality does not affect the PV of Government School Boys Adolescents. **Gupta (1992)** found that academic satisfaction was significantly related to their personalities need and personal values. The rural areas of Dehradun district are very near to the urban areas. Hence the educational environment of government schools in rural and urban areas are similar. Therefore there is no difference in the personal values of boy adolescents from government schools in urban as well as in rural areas.

e) **Comparison between rural non- government and urban non-government girl adolescents.**

TABLE-4.80

Significance of difference between RNGSGA & UNGSGA on PV

Variables	RNGSGA		UNGSGA		t	P
	M	SD	M	SD		
PVS	134.4700	14.04427	125.4600	14.17739	4.515	.000

PV= Personal Values, RNGSGA= Rural Non-Government School Girl Adolescents &
UNGSGA= Urban Non-Government School Girl Adolescents

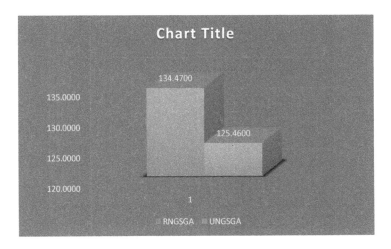

Effect of Locality on Personal Values of Non-Government School Girl Adolescents

A glance at table 4.80 reveals that the calculated t value (4.515) is significant at 0.01 level of significance (p<0.01). It means that a significant difference is found between the Personal Values of UNGSBA and UNGSGA. It also means that locality has a significant effect on PV of Non-Government School Girl Adolescents.

The mean score of RNGSGA is 134.4700 and UNGSGA is 125.4600. The mean score of RNGSGA is greater than the mean score of UNGSGA, so the result indicate that RNGSGA has more Personal Values than UNGSGA. It may be that much difference is found in the environment of non-government schools in urban and rural areas of Dehradun district. In non-government schools in urban areas, much attention is not paid on personal values but on the educational achievement of the students. Whereas in non-government schools in rural areas, personal values of the child are also developed. **Shah, H.M (1992)** showed that sex, residential area, stream of the study had significant relationship with the values of students studying in class XI and XII. Therefore the personal values of girls in rural areas of non-government schools is higher than girls in urban areas.

f) **Comparison between rural non- government and urban non-government boy adolescents.**

TABLE-4.81

Significance of difference between RNGSBA & UNGSBA on PV

Variables	RNGSBA		UNGSBA		t	P
	M	SD	M	SD		
PV	126.0700	16.83626	130.8300	15.27000	-2.094	.038

PV= Personal Values, RNGSBA= Rural Non-Government School Boy Adolescents &
UNGSBA= Urban Non-Government School Boy Adolescents

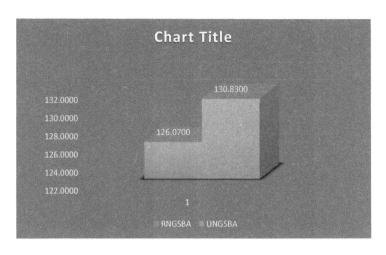

Effect of Locality on Personal Values of Non-Government School Boy Adolescents

From the content of the table 4.81 it is revealed that the calculated t value (-2.094) is significant at 0.05 level of significance (p<0.05). It means that a significant difference is found between the Personal Values of RNGSBA and UNGSBA. The mean score of RNGSBA is 126.0700 and UNGSBA is 130.8300. The mean score of UNGSBA is greater than the mean score of RNGSBA, so the result indicate that UNGSBA has more Personal Values than RNGSBA.

g) **Comparison between rural and urban government school adolescents.**

TABLE- 4.82

Significance of difference between RGSA & UGSA on PV

Variables	RGSA		UGSA		t	P
	M	SD	M	SD		
PV	135.9900	16.80392	135.1050	15.89298	.541	.589

PV = Personal Values, RGSA= Rural Government School Adolescents & UGSA= Urban Government School Adolescents

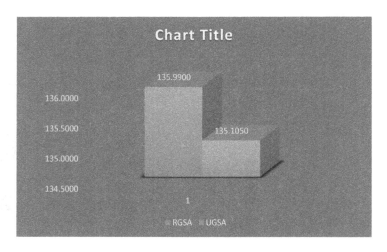

Effect of Locality on Personal Values of Government School Adolescents

A glance at table 4.82 reveals that the calculated t value (.541) is not significant at 0.05 level of significance (p>0.05). It means that there exist no significant difference between RGSA and UGSA on PV.

It shows that locality does not effect on the PV of Government School Adolescents. As we f government school in rural as well as in urban areas.

h) **Comparison between rural and urban non-government adolescents.**

TABLE- 4.83

Significance of difference between RNGSA & UNGSA on PV

Variables	RNGSA		UNGSA		t	P
	M	SD	M	SD		
PV	130.2700	16.07721	128.1450	14.94122	1.372	.171

PV= Personal Values, RNGSA= Rural Non-Government School Adolescents &
UNGSA= Urban Non-Government School Adolescents

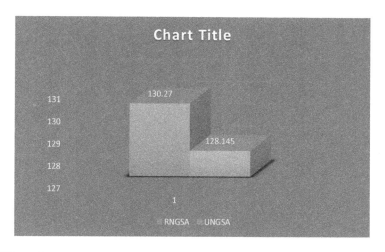

Effect of Locality on Personal Values of Non-Government School Adolescents

A careful inspection of table 4.83 revels that the calculated t value (1.372) is not significant at 0.05 level of significance (p>0.05). It means that there exist no significant difference between RNGSA and UNGSA on PV.

It show that locality has no effect on the PV of Non-Government School Adolescents. From table 4.87 we found that the personal values of RNGSGA are better than that of UNGSGA whereas from table 4.88 we found that UNGSBA have better personal values then RNGSBA. But in total there is no significance difference between the personal values of rural and urban non-government school adolescents.

i) **Comparison between rural and urban adolescents.**

TABLE- 4.84

Significance of difference between RA & UA on PV

Variables	RA		UA		t	P
	M	SD	M	SD		
PV	133.1300	16.64770	131.6250	15.79424	1.312	0.190

PV- Personal Values, RA= Rural Adolescents & UA= Urban Adolescents

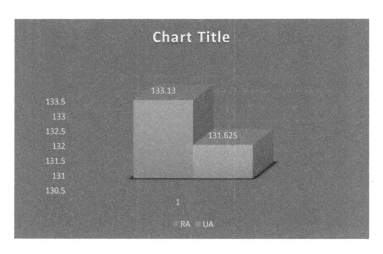

Effect of Locality on Personal Values of adolescents.

A careful inspection of table 4.84 reveals that the calculated t value (1.312) is not significant at 0.05 level of significance (p>0.05). It means that there exist no significant difference between RA and UA on PV.

It shows that locality does not affect the PV of Adolescents. It may be that the family's influence on the child's personal values are more than that of the society. Parents' Education and income affect the values of the child. **Jafri, Bilkis Sultana (1992)** revealed that there is a significant difference in the aspiration and values between high and low educated parental groups as well as between high and low parental income groups.

In rural areas of Dehradun district, SES of families differ just like families in urban areas, who try to provide healthy environment to their children. Therefore no differences has been found in the personal values of adolescent in urban and rural areas.

On the basis of above findings given in table 4.58 to 4.84 the null hypothesis VII, predicting that **"Locality does not affect self-confidence, mental health and personal values of adolescents."** is accepted and we can say that Locality has non-significant effect on self-confidence, mental health and personal values of adolescents.

PHASE VIII (A)-To find out the effect of Gender on the Self-Confident of adolescents.

a) **Comparison between rural girl and boy adolescents.**

TABLE- 4.85

Significance of difference between RBA & RGA on SC

Variables	RBA		RGA		T	P
	M	SD	M	SD		
SC	25.6750	10.13424	24.1900	9.74158	1.494	.136

SC= Self- Confidence, RBA= Rural Boy Adolescents &RGA= Rural Girl Adolescents

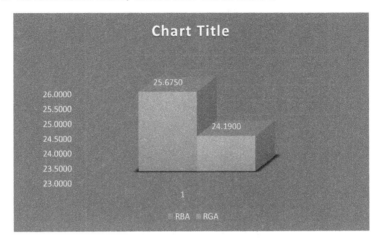

Effect of Gender on Self Confident of Rural Adolescents

A glance at table 4.85 clearly reveals that the calculated t value (1.494) is not significant at 0.05 level of significance (p>0.05). It means that there exist no significant difference between RBA and RGA on SC. It show that Gender has no effect on the SC of Rural Adolescents.

The reason for this may be that in the present study most of the rural areas of Dehradun district are peri-urban where adolescents get almost all the facilities like in urban areas. Being a semi urban area, the people here are also open minded. Like in urban areas, there is no discrimination between boys and girls in rural areas. Parents encourage both boys and girls equally, towards progress in life. Equal opportunities are provided to both and this encouragement boosts their confidence. **Geetika (2017)** found a positive relation in parental encouragement and self-confidence among adolescents. Therefore there is no difference between the self-confidence of rural boy and girl adolescents.

b) **Comparison between urban girl and boy adolescents.**

TABLE- 4.86

Significance of difference between UBA & UGA on SC

Variables	UBA		UGA		t	P
	M	SD	M	SD		
SC	25.2650	10.21354	27.5750	9.30037	-2.365	.019

SC= Self- Confidence, UBA=Urban Boy Adolescents &UGA= Urban Girl Adolescents

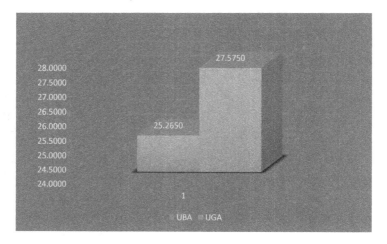

Effect of Gender on Self Confident of Urban Adolescents

A Carefully inspection of Table 4.86 reveals that the calculated t value (-2.365) which is significant at 0.05 level of significance (p<0.05). It means that a significant difference is found between the self-confidence of UBA and UGA on SC. It shows that Gender has a significant effect on SC of the Urban Adolescents.

The mean score of UBA is 25.2650 and UGA is 27.5750. The mean score of UGA is greater than the mean score of UBA, in the present study more self-confidence score means less self-confidence and less self-confidence score means more self-confidence.

So the result indicate that UBA has more confidence than UGA.

It could be due to the innate biological differences present between both the genders. Boys are stronger than girls. They are not afraid to do any work and this power boosts their confidence. **Ziegler et. al. (2000)** reported that girls expressed significantly lower level of self-confidence than boys.

c) **Comparison between rural government girl and boy adolescents.**

TABLE- 4.87

Significance of difference between RGSBA & RGSGA on SC

Variables	RGSBA		RGSGA		T	P
	M	SD	M	SD		
SC	25.0500	10.71521	26.3100	10.37742	-.845	.399

SC= Self- Confidence, RGSBA=Rural Government School Boy Adolescents
RGSGA= Rural Government School Girl Adolescents

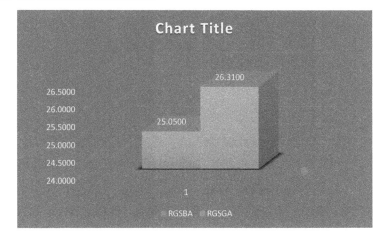

Effect of Gender on Self Confident of Rural Government School Adolescents

A careful inspection of Table 4.87 reveals that the calculated t value (-.845) is not significant at 0.05 level of significance (p>0.05). It means that there exist no significant difference between RGSBA and RGSGA on SC. It show that Gender has no effect on the SC of Rural Government School Adolescents.

It shows that both RGSGA and RGSBA are equally self-confident. The reason for this may be that there is no difference in the self-confidence of boys and girls studying in government schools in rural areas due to being in the same area and studying in similar type of school environment. **Ghaonta (2015)** found that male and female school students possess almost equal level of self-confidence.

d) **Comparison between urban government girl and boy adolescents.**

TABLE- 4.88

Significance of difference between UGSBA & UGSGA on SC

Variables	UGSBA		UGSGA		t	P
	M	SD	M	SD		

| SC | 26.8000 | 10.39522 | 28.0800 | 9.61237 | -.904 | .367 |

SC= Self- Confidence, UGSBA= Urban Government School Boy Adolescents
UGSGA= Urban Government School Girl Adolescents

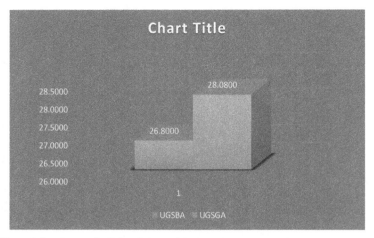

Effect of Gender on Self Confident of Urban Government School Adolescents

A glance at table 4.88 reveals that the calculated t value (-.904) is not significant at 0.05 level of significance (p>0.05). It means that there exist no significant difference between UGSBA and UGSGA on SC.

It shows that Gender has no effect on the SC of Urban Government School Adolescents. As we know, there is no discrimination between boys and girls in urban areas. Both have a freedom to express their thought. Therefore due to studying in the same type of school environment there is no significant difference between the self-confidence in them. **Wankhade and Rokade (2011)** also found that the self-confidence of both sexes from urban areas are almost same.

e) **Comparison between rural non- government girl and boy adolescents.**

TABLE- 4.89

Significance of difference between RNGSBA & RNGSGA on SC

Variables	RNGSBA		RNGSGA		t	P
	M	SD	M	SD		
SC	26.3000	9.53092	22.0700	8.60145	3.295	.001

SC= Self- Confidence, RNGSBA=Rural Non- Government School Boy Adolescents
RNGSGA= Rural Non-Government School Girl Adolescents

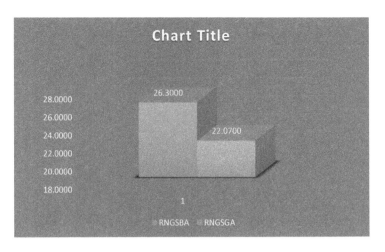

Effect of Gender on Self Confident of Rural Non- Government School Adolescents

From the content of table 4.89 it is revealed that the calculated t value (3.295) is significant at 0.01 level of significance (p<0.01).It means that a significant difference is found between the self-confidence of RNGSBA and RNGSGA. It also means that Gender has a significant effect on SC of Rural Non-Government School Adolescents. The mean score of RNGSBA is 26.3000 and RNGSGA is 22.0700. The mean score of RNGSBA is greater than the mean score of RNGSGA, in the present study more self-confidence score means less confidence and less self-confidence score means more confident. So the result indicate that RNGSGA has more confident than RNGSBA.

The result is in congruence with **Lal Krishan (2014)** who found that female adolescents are high on self-confidence in comparison to male adolescents.

f) **Comparison between urban non- government girl and boy adolescents.**

Table- 4.90

Significance of difference between UNGSBA & UNGSGA on SC

Variables	UNGSBA		UNGSGA		t	P
	M	SD	M	SD		
SC	23.7300	9.84204	27.0700	8.99748	-2.505	.013

SC= Self- Confidence, UNGSBA= Urban Non-Government School Boy Adolescents

UNGSGA= Urban Non-Government School Girl Adolescents

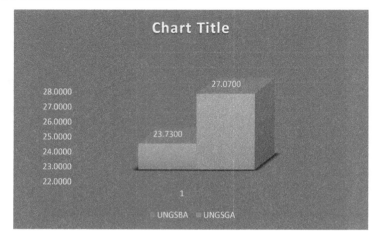

Effect of Gender on Self Confident of Urban Non- Government School Adolescents

Table 4.90 reveals that the calculated t value (-2.505) is significant at 0.05 level of significance (p<0.05). It means that a significant difference is found between the self-confidence of UNGSBA and UNGSGA. It shows that Gender has a significant effect on SC of Urban Non-Government School Adolescents. The mean score of UNGSBA is 23.7300 and UNGSGA is 27.0700. The mean score of UNGSGA is greater than the mean score of UNGSBA, in the present study more self-confidence score means less confident and less self-confidence score means more confident so the result indicate that UNGSBA has more confident than UNGSGA.

The reason for this may be that, in non-government schools in urban areas the emphasis is on students to score more. Girls are more sincere than boys. Girls take more stress of studies than boys and **Selvaraj and Gnanadevan (2014)** found that there is a significant and negative relationship between self-confidence and different dimension of stress such as academic stress, interpersonal stress, intrapersonal stress, Environmental stress and total stress. This means those who take more stress are less confident. Therefore the self-confidence of girls from non-government school in urban areas is lower than the self-confidence of boys.

g) **Comparison between government school girl and boy adolescents.**

TABLE- 4.91

Significance of difference between GSBA & GSGA on SC

Variables	GSBA	GSGA	t	P

	M	SD	M	SD		
SC	25.9250	10.56634	27.1950	10.01642	-1.234	.218

SC= Self- Confidence, GSBA=Government School Boy Adolescents
GSGA= Government School Girl Adolescents

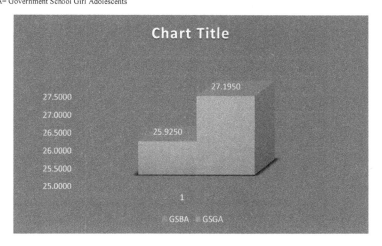

Effect of Gender on Self Confident of Government School Adolescents

A study of table 4.91reveals that the calculated t value (-1.234) is not significant at 0.05 level of significance (p>0.05).It means that there exist no significant difference between GSBA and GSGA on SC. It show that Gender has no effect on the SC of Government School Adolescents.

The reason could be that in table 4.94 we found no difference in the self-confidence of boys and girls studying in government schools in rural areas also from table 4.95 we found that there is no difference in the self-confidence of urban girls and boys studying in government school. Therefore as a whole, no difference has been found in the self-confidence of boys and girls studying in government school.

h) **Comparison between non- government school girl and boy adolescents.**

TABLE- 4.92

Significance of difference between NGSBA & NGSGA on SC

Variables	NGSBA		NGSGA		t	P
	M	SD	M	SD		
SC	25.0150	9.74884	24.5700	9.13027	.471	.638

SC= Self- Confidence, NGSBA= Non-Government School Boy Adolescents

NGSGA= Non-Government School Girl Adolescents

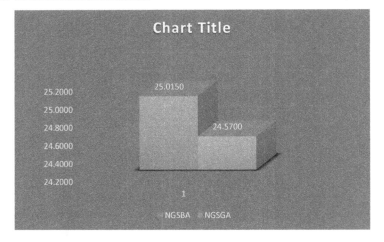

Effect of Gender on Self -Confident of Non-Government School Adolescents

A perusal of table 4.92reveals that the calculated t value (.471) is not significant at 0.05 level of significance (p>0.05).It means that there exist no significant difference between NGSBA and NGSGA on SC. It show that Gender has no effect on the SC of Non-Government School Adolescents.

i) **Comparison between girl and boy adolescents.**

TABLE- 4.93

Significance of difference between BA & GA on SC

Variables	BA		GA		t	P
	M	SD	M	SD		
SC	25.4700	10.16328	25.8825	9.66137	-.588	.556

SC= Self- Confidence, BA=Boy Adolescents &GA= Girl Adolescents

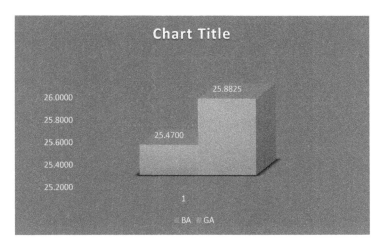

Effect of Gender on Self Confident of Adolescents

A perusal of table 4.93 reveals that the calculated t value (-.588) is not significant at 0.05 level of significance (p>0.05). It means that there exist no significant difference between BA and GA on SC. It shows that Gender does not affect the SC of Adolescents.

The finding is in congruence with the study made by **Dr. Meena Sharma (2015)** revealing that the two groups (Male & Female) did not differ significantly in self – Confidence. **Verma, R.K. and kumara Saroj (2016)** also reported that there were no significant difference in the self- confidence of male and female elementary school students.

PHASE VIII (B)-To find out the effect of gender on the mental health of adolescents.

a) **Comparison between rural girl and boy adolescents.**

TABLE- 4.94

Significance of difference between RBA & RGA on MH

Variables	RBA		RGA		t	P
	M	SD	M	SD		
MH	74.6050	10.47222	77.1700	9.08094	-2.617	.009

MH= Mental Health, RBA= Rural Boy Adolescents &RGA= Rural Girl Adolescents

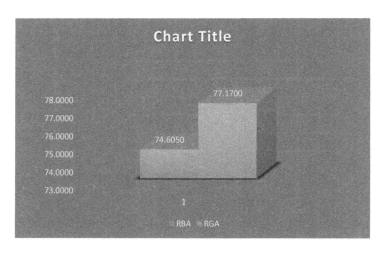

Effect of Gender on Mental Health of Rural Adolescents

A perusal of Table 4.94 reveals that the calculated t value (-2.617) is significant at 0.05 level of significance (p<0.05). It means that a significant difference is found between the Mental Health of RBA and RGA. The mean score of RBA is 74.6050 and RGA is 77.1700. The mean score of RGA is greater than the mean score of RBA, so the result indicate that RGA has more Mental Health than RBA.

It shows that in rural area Gender has a significant effect on MH. The reason could be that since girls tend to be more emotionally stable in relationship as compared to boys, their adjustment level is higher than that of the boys. **Mehta et. al., (2005)** has also found that girls were better adjusted than boys and **Srividhya, V. and Khadi, Pushpa, B. (2007)** found that mental health was significantly correlated to adjustment problem, indicating higher the problem lower the mental health.

That is, one who has a low level of adjustment his mental health is also low and because the adjustment level of girls is higher than boys therefore their mental health is also better than that of boys.

b) **Comparison between urban girl and boy adolescents.**

TABLE- 4.95

Significance of difference between UBA & UGA on MH

Variables	UBA		UGA		t	P
	M	SD	M	SD		
MH	75.4300	10.79294	74.8400	9.13299	.590	.555

MH= Mental Health, UBA= Urban Boy Adolescents &UGA= Urban Girl Adolescents

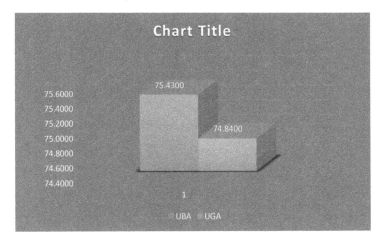

Effect of Gender on Mental Health of Urban Adolescents

A careful inspection of Table 4.95 reveals that the calculated t value (.590) is not significant at 0.05 level of significance (p>0.05). It means that there exist no significant difference between UBA and UGA on MH.

It shows that in urban area Gender has no effect on the MH. The finding is supported by **Mittal. A. (2008)** who found that the mental health of secondary level of student of urban localities are same.

c) **Comparison between rural government girl and boy adolescents.**

TABLE- 4.96

Significance of difference between RGSBA & RGSGA on MH

Variables	RGSBA		RGSGA		T	P
	M	SD	M	SD		
MH	76.0600	11.19598	77.8600	10.21785	-1.188	.236

MH= Mental Health, RGSBA=Rural Government School Boy Adolescents
RGSGA= Rural Government School Girl Adolescents

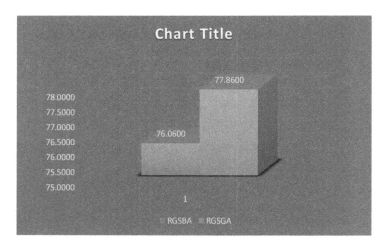

Effect of Gender on Mental Health of Rural Government School Adolescents

A perusal of Table 4.96 reveals that the calculated t value (-1.188) is not significant at 0.05 level of significance (p>0.05). It means that there exist no significant difference between RGSBA and RGSGA on MH.

It shows that Gender does not affect the MH of Rural Government School Adolescents. **Mittal. A. (2008)** found that the mental health of secondary school student of rural localities are same. Therefore due to studying in the same school environment no different has been found in the mental health of boy and girl adolescents from government school of rural areas.

d) **Comparison between urban government School girl and boy adolescents.**

TABLE- 4.97

Significance of difference between UGSBA & UGSGA on MH

Variables	UGSBA		UGSGA		t	P
	M	SD	M	SD		
MH	75.9400	11.48457	77.2200	8.44899	-.898	.370

MH= Mental Health, UGSBA= Urban Government School Boy Adolescents
UGSGA= Urban Government School Girl Adolescents

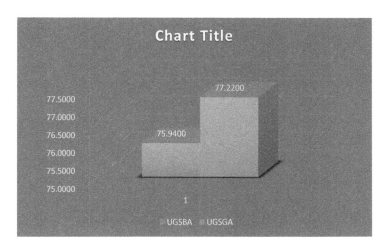

Effect of Gender on Mental Health of Urban Government School Adolescents

A glance at Table 4.97 reveals that the calculated t value (-.898) is not significant at 0.05 level of significance (p>0.05). It means that there exist no significant difference between UGSBA and UGSGA on MH.

It shows that Gender does not affect the MH of Urban Government School Adolescents. **Mittal. A. (2008)** found that the mental health of secondary school student of urban localities are same. Therefore due to studying in the same school environment no different has been found in the mental health of boy and girl adolescents from government school of urban areas.

e) **Comparison between rural non- government School girl and boy adolescents.**

TABLE- 4.98

Significance of difference between RNGSBA & RNGSGA on MH

Variables	RNGSBA		RNGSGA		T	P
	M	SD	M	SD		
MH	73.1500	9.52972	76.4800	7.77133	-2.708	.007

MH= Mental Health, RNGSBA=Rural Non- Government School Boy Adolescents
RNGSGA= Rural Non-Government School Girl Adolescents

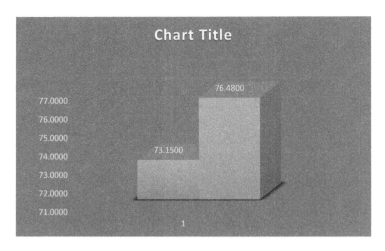

Effect of Gender on Mental Health of Rural Non- Government School Adolescents

A perusal of table 4.98reveals that the calculated t value (-2.708) is significant at 0.05 level of significance (p<0.05).It means that a significant difference is found between the Mental Health of RNGSBA and RNGSGA. It also means that Gender has a significant effect on MH of Rural Non-Government School Adolescents. The mean score of RNGSBA is 73.1500 and RNGSGA is 76.4800. The mean score of RNGSGA is greater than the mean score of RNGSBA, so the result indicate that RNGSGA has more Mental Health than RNGSBA.

It could be because girls are more adjustive than boys and girls are also emotionally stable. Adjustability and emotion stability may be helpful in enhancing their mental health. The result is in congruence with **Mehta et. al., (2005)** who found that were girls better adjusted then boys. **Dr. Chitra (2017)** found that private school girls are more emotionally stable then the private school boys. **Srividhya, V. and Khadi, Pushpa, B. (2007)** also confirmed that mental health was significantly correlated to adjustment problems indicating higher the problem lower the mental health. And **Hay and Ashman (2003)** also confirmed that emotional stability may be cited as calmness of mind and freedom from anxiety and depression.

f) **Comparison between urban non- government girl and boy adolescents.**

Table- 4.99

Significance of difference between UNGSBA & UNGSGA on MH

Variables	UNGSBA		UNGSGA		t	P
	M	SD	M	SD		
MH	74.9200	10.08617	72.4600	9.21069	1.801	.073

MH= Mental Health, UNGSBA= Urban Non-Government School Boy Adolescents
UNGSGA= Urban Non-Government School Girl Adolescents

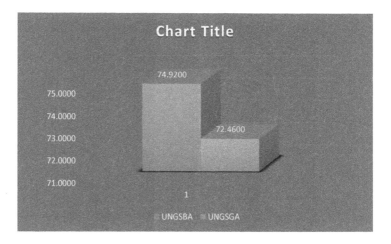

Effect of Gender on Mental Health of Urban Non- Government School Adolescents

A glance at table 4.99 clearly reveals that the calculated t value (1.801) which is not significant at 0.05 level of significance (p>0.05). It means that there exist no significant difference between UNGSBA and UNGSGA on MH. It show that Gender has no effect on the MH of Urban Non-Government School Adolescents.

This may be due to the fact that there is no difference in the mental health of boys and girls studying in non-government schools in urban areas due to studying in similar school environment and living in the same areas. **Sarita, Dahiya, Rajni and Pushpanjali (2015)** also found that the mental health of boys and girls of private senior secondary schools are same.

g) **Comparison between government school girl and boy adolescents.**

TABLE- 4.100

Significance of difference between GSBA & GSGA on MH

Variables	GSBA		GSGA		t	P
	M	SD	M	SD		
MH	76.0000	11.31282	77.5400	9.35715	-1.483	0.139

MH= Mental Health, GSBA=Government School Boy Adolescents
GSGA= Government School Girl Adolescents

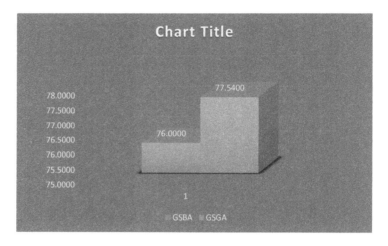

Effect of Gender on Mental Health of Government School Adolescents

A careful inspection of table 4.100 reveals that the calculated t value is (-1.483) is not significant at 0.05 level of significance (p>0.05). It means that there exist no significant difference between GSBA and GSGA on MH. It also means that Gender has no effect on MH of Government School Adolescents.

This may be because no difference has been found in the mental health of boys and girls of Government school due to studying in the similar school environment. The finding is in congruence with the study made by **Sarita, Dahiya Rajni, and Puspanjali (2015)** who revealed that the mental health of boys and girls of government senior secondary schools are same.

h) **Comparison between non- government school girl and boy adolescents.**

TABLE- 4.101

Significance of difference between NGSBA & NGSGA on MH

Variables	NGSBA		NGSGA		t	P
	M	SD	M	SD		
MH	74.0350	9.82734	74.4700	8.73560	-.468	.640

MH= Mental Health, NGSBA= Non-Government School Boy Adolescents
NGSGA= Non-Government School Girl Adolescents

Effect of Gender on Mental Health of Non-Government School Adolescents

A statistical analysis of table 4.101 indicates that the calculated t value (-.468) is not significant at 0.05 level of significance (p>0.05). It means that there exist no significant difference between NGSBA and NGSGA on MH. It show that Gender has no effect on the MH of Non-Government School Adolescents.

The result is in congruence with findings of **Anju (2000) who** found that emotional maturity level of the senior secondary school students (boys and girls) of the Chandigarh is almost same and **Sarita, Dahiya, Rajni and Pushpanjali (2015)** also found that the mental health of boys and girls of private senior secondary schools are same.

i) Comparison between girl and boy adolescents.

TABLE-4.102

Significance of difference between BA & GA on MH

Variables	BA		GA		T	P
	M	SD	M	SD		
MH	75.0175	10.62848	76.0050	9.17007	-1.407	.160

MH= Mental Health, BA= Boy Adolescents &GA= Girl Adolescents

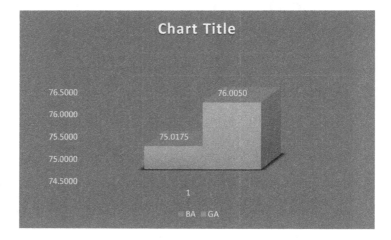

Effect of Gender on Mental Health of Adolescents

A glance at table 4.102 reveals that the calculated t value (-1.407) is not significant at 0.05 level of significance (p>0.05).It means that there exist no significant difference between BA and GA on MH.

It shows that Gender has no effect on the MH of Adolescents. The finding are supported by **Srividhya, V.; and Khadi, Pushpa, B. (2007)** who found that boys and girls did not differ in mental health state. **Singh, B., Kumar, A. and Moral, A. (2015)** also found that there is no significant difference between the mental health of male and female students.

PHASE VIII (C)-To find out the effect of gender on the personal values of adolescents.

a) **Comparison between rural girl and boy adolescents.**

TABLE- 4.103

Significance of difference between RBA & RGA on PV

Variables	RBA		RGA		T	P
	M	SD	M	SD		
PV	130.0150	17.57925	136.2450	15.07152	-3.805	0.00

PV= Personal Values, RBA= Rural Boy Adolescents &RGA= Rural Girl Adolescents

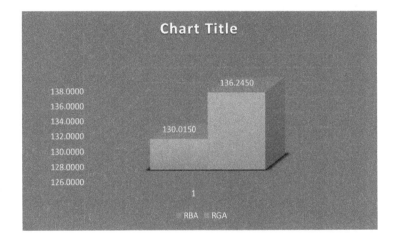

Effect of Gender on Personal Values of Rural Adolescents

A perusal at Table 4.103 reveals that the calculated t value (-3.805) is significant at 0.01 level of significance (p<0.01). It means that a significant difference is found between the Personal Values of RBA and RGA. It shows that Gender has a significant effect on PV of Rural Adolescents.

The mean score of RBA is 130.0150 and RGA is 136.2450. The mean score of RGA is greater than the mean score of RBA, so the result indicate that RGA has more Personal Values than RBA. In rural areas girls spend most of their time at home, so more attention is paid to the development of values in girls than boys. Girls are given household responsibilities. Due to which personal values like honesty, love, cleanliness, discipline etc. develop on their own. Therefore the personal values of girls in rural areas is higher than boys.

b) Comparison between urban girl and boy adolescents.

TABLE- 4.104

Significance of difference between UBA & UGA on PV

Variables	UBA		UGA		T	P
	M	SD	M	SD		
PV	132.2300	17.37806	131.0200	14.05122	.766	.444

PV= Personal Values, UBA= Urban Boy Adolescents &UGA= Urban Girl Adolescents

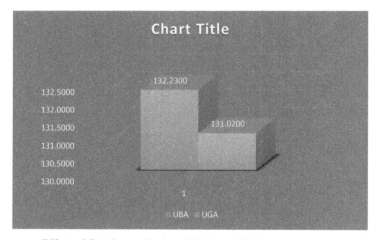

Effect of Gender on Personal Values of Urban Adolescents

A careful inspection of Table 4.104 reveals that the calculated t value (.766) is not significant at 0.05 level of significance (p>0.05). It means that there exist no significant difference between UBA and UGA on PV.

It shows that Gender does not affect the PV of urban Adolescents. It may be that in urban areas parents provide a similar environment to both boys and girls. Girls are provided with the same freedom as boys. Hence no difference has been found in the personal values of the two due to a common environment.

c) **Comparison between rural government girl and boy adolescents.**

TABLE- 4.105

Significance of difference between RGSBA & RGSGA on PV

Variables	RGSBA		RGSGA		T	P
	M	SD	M	SD		
PV	133.9600	17.50089	138.0200	15.90564	-1.717	.088

PV= Personal Values, RGSBA= Rural Government School Boy Adolescents
RGSGA= Rural Government School Girl Adolescents

Chart Title

- RGSBA: 133.9600
- RGSGA: 138.0200

Effect of Gender on Personal Values of Rural Government School Adolescents

A Statistical analysis of table 4.105 indicates that the calculated t value (-1.717) is not significant at 0.05 level of significance (p>0.05).It means that there exist no significant difference between RGSBA and RGSGA on PV. It show that Gender has no effect on the PV of Rural Government School Adolescents.

The reason for this may be that the people of rural areas are very simple in nature. They have a feeling of love and cooperation towards each other and they are honest. They transfer all the feeling to their children also. **Blais (2010)** also found that personal values will be developed through being influenced by family, culture society, environment, religious belief and Ethnicity. Therefore there is no difference in the personal values of boys and girls studying in government schools in rural areas.

d) Comparison between urban government School girl and boy adolescents.

TABLE- 4.106

Significance of difference between UGSBA & UGSGA on PV

Variables	UGSBA		UGSGA		t	P
	M	SD	M	SD		
PV	133.6300	19.23310	136.5800	11.55066	-1.315	.190

PV= Personal Values, UGSBA= Urban Government School Boy Adolescents
UGSGA= Urban Government School Girl Adolescents

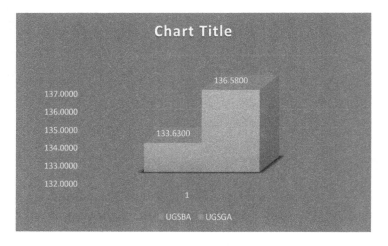

Effect of Gender on Personal Values of Urban Government School Adolescents

A careful inspection of table 4.106 reveals that the calculated t value (-1.315) is not significant at 0.05 level of significance (p>0.05). It means that there exist no significant difference between UGSBA and UGSGA on PV. It show that Gender has no effect on the PV of Urban Government School Adolescents.

The reason for this could be that both boys and girls are effected by the pomp and show of urban life. And because the school environment is also similar, no difference has been found in the personal values of boys and girls studying in government schools or urban areas.

e) **Comparison between rural non- government School girl and boy adolescents.**

TABLE- 4.107

Significance of difference between RNGSBA & RNGSGA on PV

Variables	RNGSBA		RNGSGA		T	P
	M	SD	M	SD		
PVS	126.0700	16.83626	134.4700	14.04427	-3.831	.000

PV= Personal Values, RNGSBA=Rural Non- Government School Boy Adolescents
RNGSGA= Rural Non-Government School Girl Adolescents

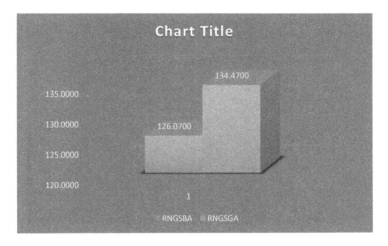

Effect of Gender on Personal Values of Rural Non- Government School Adolescents

A perusal of table 4.107reveals that the calculated t value (-3.831) is significant at 0.05 level of significance (p<0.05).It means that a significant difference is found between the Personal Values of RNGSBA and RNGSGA. It also means that Gender has a significant effect on PV of Rural Non-Government School Adolescents. The mean score of RNGSBA is 126.0700 and RNGSGA is 134.7400. The mean score of RNGSGA is greater than the mean score of RNGSBA, so the result indicate that RNGSGA has more Personal Values than RNGSBA.

The above result is in congruence with the finding **Dr. Mamta (2017)** who found that the female students have high moral values then male students of secondary school.

Dr. Bhutiya (2013) also found that gender plays a significant role in the personal values of adolescents.

f) Comparison between urban non- government girl and boy adolescents.

Table- 4.108

Significance of difference between UNGSBA & UNGSGA on PV

Variables	UNGSBA		UNGSGA		t	P
	M	SD	M	SD		
PV	130.8300	15.27000	125.4600	14.17739	2.577	.011

PV= Personal Values, UNGSBA=Urban Non-Government School Boy Adolescents
UNGSGA= Urban Non-Government School Girl Adolescents

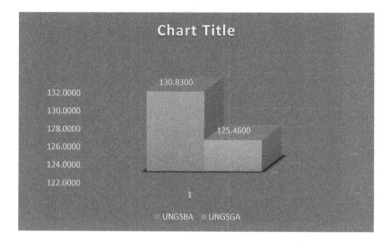

Effect of Gender on Personal Values of Urban Non- Government School Adolescents

The statistically calculated t value (2.577) is significant at 0.05 level of significance ($p<0.05$). It means that a significant difference is found between the Personal Values of UNGSBA and UNGSGA. It also means that Gender has a significant effect on PV of Urban Non-Government School Adolescents.

The mean score of UNGSBA is 130.8300 and UNGSGA is 125.4600. The mean score of UNGSBA is greater than the mean score of UNGSGA, so the result indicate that UNGSBA has more Personal Values than UNGSGA.

g) **Comparison between government school girl and boy adolescents.**

TABLE- 4.109

Significance of difference between GSBA & GSGA on PV

Variables	GSBA		GSGA		t	P
	M	SD	M	SD		
PV	133.7950	18.34189	137.3000	13.88358	-2.155	.032

PV= Personal Values, GSBA=Government School Boy Adolescents
GSGA= Government School Girl Adolescents

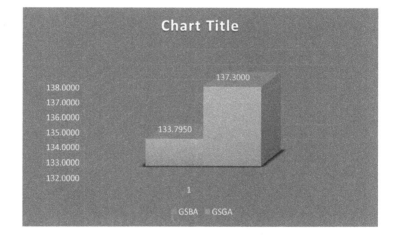

Effect of Gender on Personal Values of Government School Adolescents

The perusal of table 4.109 reveals that the calculated t value (-2.155) is significant at 0.05 level of significance (p<0.05). It means that a significant difference is found between the Personal Values of GSBA and GSGA. It show that Gender has a significant effect on the PV of Government School Adolescents. The mean score of GSBA is 133.7850 and GSGA is 137.3000. The mean score of GSGA is greater than the mean score of GSBA, so the result indicate that GSGA has good personal values than GSBA.

The reason for this may be that even today in Indian society, emphasis is placed on making girls more valuable than boys. **Dr. Mamta Taneja (2017)** also found that female students have high moral values than male students of secondary school. That is why the personal values of girls is good than that of boys even though they are studying in the similar school.

h) **Comparison between non- government school girl and boy adolescents.**

TABLE- 4.110

Significance of difference between NGSBA & NGSGA on PV

Variables	NGSBA		NGSGA		T	P
	M	SD	M	SD		
PV	128.4500	16.20836	129.9650	14.78230	-.977	0.329

PV= Personal Values, NGSBA= Non-Government School Boy Adolescents
NGSGA= Non-Government School Girl Adolescents

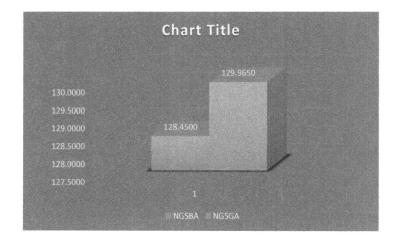

Effect of Gender on Personal Values of Non-Government School Adolescents

The statistically calculated t value (-.977) is not significant at 0.05 level (p>0.05). It means that there exist no significant difference between NGSBA and NGSGA on PV. It shows that gender has no effect on the PV of Non-Government school adolescents

i) **Comparison between girl and boy adolescents.**

TABLE-4.111

Significance of difference between BA & GA on PV

Variables	BA		GA		T	P
	M	SD	M	SD		

| PV | 131.1225 | 17.49221 | 133.6325 | 14.78526 | -2.192 | .029 |

PV= Personal Values, BA=Boy Adolescents &GA= Girl Adolescents

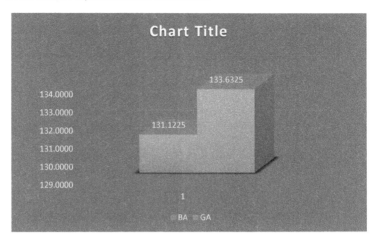

Effect of Gender on Personal Values of Adolescents

A glance at Table 4.111 reveals that the calculated t value (- 2.192) is significant at 0.05 level of significance (p<0.05).It means that a significant difference is found between the Personal Values of BA and GA. It shows that Gender has a significant effect on PV of Adolescents.

The mean score of BA is 131.1225 and GA is 133.6325. The mean score of GA is greater than the mean score of BA, so the result indicate that GA has more Personal Values than BA. This may be due to differences in the tendencies of boys and girls. Girls are more honest and helpful than boys. They adopt good habits. They have more sense of affection than boys. They are more disciplined **Ismail, H.(2015)** also found that females plays a higher weight on personal values related to the broad categories of "Ethics" and "citizenship", while males put a stronger emphasis on "masculinity". Therefore the girl adolescents have highest personal values than boys.

Thus, result obtained from Tables 4.85 to 4.111clarifies that Gender has non-significant effect on self-confidence and mental health but a significant effect on personal values of adolescents. So the VIII hypothesis predicting **"No significant difference are obtained between self-confidence, mental health and personal values of adolescents when comparison is made on the basis of gender." Is** only partially accepted.

PHASE IX (A)- To find out the effect of types of school on the self- confidence of adolescents.

a) **Comparison between government school and non-government school girl adolescents.**

TABLE- 4.112

Significance of difference between GSGA & NGSGA on SC

Variables	GSGA		NGSGA		t	P
	M	SD	M	SD		
SC	27.1950	10.01642	24.5700	9.13027	2.739	.006

SC= Self-Confidence, GSGA= Government School Girl Adolescents, NGSGA= Non-Government School Girl Adolescents

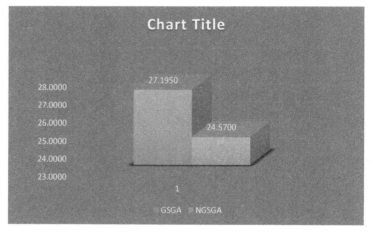

Effect of types of school on Self Confidence of Girls Adolescents

Table 4.112, reveals that the calculated t value (2.739) is significant at 0.01 level of significance (p<0.01). It means that a significant difference is found between the self-confidence of GSGA and NGSGA. It shows that types of School has a significant effect on SC of Girls Adolescents. The mean score of GSGA is 27.1950 and NGSGA is 24.5700. The mean score of GSGA is greater than the mean score of NGSGA, in the present study more self-confidence score means less confidence and less self-confidence score means more confident. So the result indicate that NGSGA has more confident than GGSA.

The reason for this may be that most of the students who study in non-government schools have high SES. Adolescent girls spend most of their time either at home or in school. Therefore girls studying in non-government schools get a healthy environment both at home as well as at school. Which boosts their self-confidence. Whereas most of the students studying in government schools have low SES, due to which they are not able to get such an environment both at home and school which can increase their self-confidence. Therefore the self-confidence of girls of non-government schools are higher than the girls from government school.

b) **Comparison between government school and non-government school boy adolescents.**

TABLE- 4.113

Significance of difference between GSBA & NGSBA on SC

Variables	GSBA		NGSBA		t	P
	M	SD	M	SD		
SC	25.9250	10.56634	25.0150	9.74884	.895	.371

SC= Self-Confidence, GSBA= Government School Boy Adolescents, NGSBA= Non-Government School Boy Adolescents

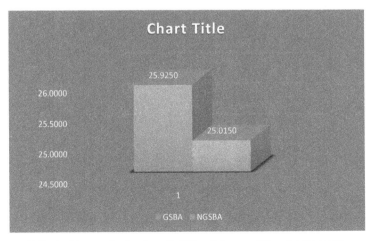

Effect of types of school on Self Confidence of Boy Adolescents

A careful inspection of Table 4.113 reveals that the calculated t value (.895) is not significant at 0.05 level of significance (p>0.05). It means that there exist no significant difference between GSBA and NGSBA on SC. It shows that type of school does not effect on the SC of Boy Adolescents.

It may be that in Indian society, boys have the freedom to do any task fearlessly. Both the society and the family provide them the freedom to do every work. No restriction is imposed on them which keeps their confidence. Therefore the type of school has no effect on their self-confidence.

c) **Comparison between rural government and non-government school girl adolescents.**

TABLE- 4.114

Significance of difference between RGSGA & RNGSGA on SC

Variables	RGSGA		RNGSGA		T	P
	M	SD	M	SD		
SC	26.3100	10.37742	22.0700	8.60145	3.146	.002

SC= Self-Confidence, RGSGA= Rural Government School Girl Adolescents,
RNGSGA= Rural Non-Government School Girl Adolescents

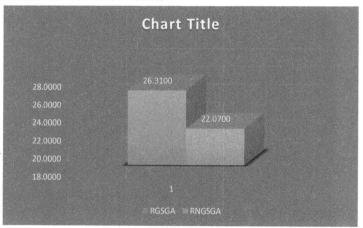

Effect of types of school on Self Confidence of Rural Girl Adolescents

A study of table 4.114 reveals that the calculated t value (3.146) is significant at 0.01 level of significance (p<0.01).It means that a significant difference is found between the self-confidence of RGSGA and RNGSGA on SC. It shows that types of School has a significant effect on SC of Rural Girl Adolescents. The mean score of RGSGA is 26.3100 and RNGSGA is 22.0700. The mean score of RGSGA is greater than the mean score of RNGSGA, in the present study more self-confidence score means less confidence and less self-confidence score means more confident. So the result indicate that RNGSGA has more confident than RGSGA.

The reason for this may be that girls tend to be shy in nature. Even today in Indian society girls are not given full freedom as compared to boys. But school is a place where everyone is provided equal opportunities for development the school environment plays a significant role in the development of different personality traits in adolescents. In Non-Government schools, a consideration is also given to educational development as well as other development of children. Children are provided with various type of activities with which they are able to develop their qualities according to their interest. Which can be helpful in boosting their self-confidence. But due to lack of facilities in government schools, the overall development of the child may be affected. Therefore the confidence of girls studying in non-government schools of rural areas is higher than the confidence of girls studying in government schools of rural areas.

d) **Comparison between rural government and non-government school boy adolescents.**

TABLE- 4.115

Significance of difference between RGSBA & RNGSBA on SC

Variables	RGSBA		RNGSBA		T	P
	M	SD	M	SD		
SC	25.0500	10.71521	26.3000	9.53092	.872	.384

SC= Self-Confidence, RGSBA= Rural Government School Boy Adolescents,
RNGSBA= Rural Non-Government School Boy Adolescents

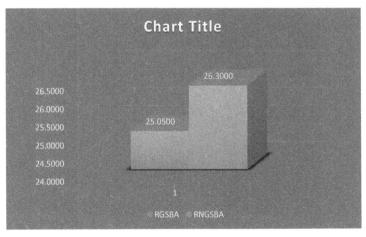

Effect of types of school on Self Confidence of Rural Boy Adolescents

A perusal of Table 4.115 reveals that the t value (.872) is not significant at 0.05 level of significance (p>0.05). It means that there exist no significant difference between RGSBA and RNGSBA on SC.

It shows that type of school does not affect the SC of Rural Boys Adolescents. This might be due to the fact that in adolescents confidence also arises from their home environment. The girls learn to be adjustive emotionally, socially and educationally from their families and carry forward the same adjustment pattern to their school. In urban areas parents do not make any difference between boys and girls. They also give girls the same freedom as boys which increases their self-confidence. So for them the type of school is no criteria for self-confidence. Therefore no difference has been found in the self-confidence of girls studying in government and non-government school in urban areas.

e) **Comparison between urban government and non-government school girl adolescents.**

TABLE- 4.116

Significance of difference between UGSGA & UNGSGA on SC

Variables	UGSGA		UNGSGA		t	P
	M	SD	M	SD		
SC	28.0800	9.61237	27.0700	8.99748	.767	.444

SC= Self-Confidence, UGSGA= Urban Government School Girl Adolescents,
UNGSGA= Urban Non-Government School Girl Adolescents

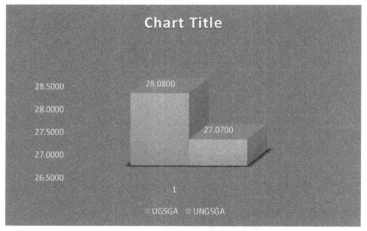

Effect of types of school on Self Confidence of Urban Girl Adolescents

A carful inspection of Table 4.116 reveals that the calculated t value (.767) which is not significant at 0.05 level of significance (p>0.05). It means that there exist no significant difference between UGSGA and UNGSGA on SC. It shows that type of school does not effect on the SC of Urban Girl Adolescents.

It could be because the urban society is influenced by technological advancements leading to change in the life style and personality of adolescents. It may also be that in urban areas, parents being open minded, they encourage their children to do everything's. They provide all kind of facilities due to which their self-confidence remains elevated. Therefore no significant difference was found in the self-confidence of girls studying in government and non-government schools in urban areas.

f) **Comparison between urban government and non-government school boy adolescents.**

TABLE- 4.117

Significance of difference between UGSBA & UNGSBA on SC

Variables	UGSBA		UNGSBA		t	P
	M	SD	M	SD		
SC	26.8000	10.39522	23.7300	9.84204	2.145	.033

SC= Self-Confidence, UGSBA= Urban Government School Boy Adolescents,
UNGSBA= Urban Non-Government School Boy Adolescents

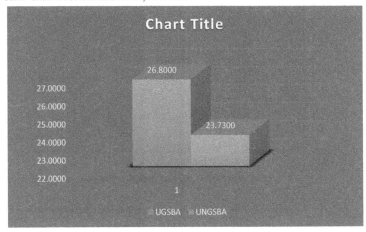

Effect of types of school on Self Confidence of Urban Boy Adolescents

The statistically calculated t value (2.145) is significant at 0.05 level of significance (p<0.05). It means that a significant difference is found between the self-confidence of UGSBA and UNGSBA on SC. It means that types of School has a significant effect on SC of Urban Boys Adolescents. The mean score of UGSBA is 26.8000 and UNGSBA is 23.7300. The mean score of UGSBA is greater than the mean score of UNGSBA, in the present study more self-confidence score means less self-confidence and low self-confidence score means more confidence. So the result indicate that UNGSBA has more Confident than UGSBA.

g) **Comparison between Rural government and non-government school adolescents.**

TABLE- 4.18

Significance of difference between RGSA & RNGSA on SC

Variables	RGSA		RNGSA		t	P
	M	SD	M	SD		
SC	25.6800	10.54007	24.1850	9.30017	1.504	.133

SC= Self-Confidence, RGSA= Rural Government School Adolescents,
RNGSA= Rural Non-Government School Adolescents

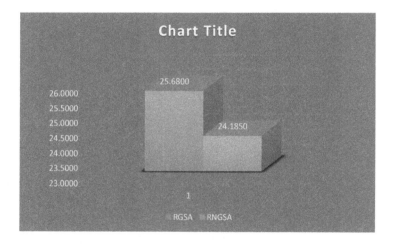

Effect of types of school on Self Confidence of Rural Adolescents

A glance of table 4.118 clearly reveals that the calculated t value (1.504) is not significant at 0.05 level of significance (p>0.05). It means that there exist no significant difference between RGSA and RNGSA on SC. It shows that type of school does not affect the SC of Rural Adolescents.

In rural government and non-government schools, there is no difference in their schools environment other than medium of instruction. Therefore no difference has been found in the self-confidence of adolescents studying there.

h) **Comparison between Urban government and non-government school adolescents.**

TABLE- 4.119

Significance of difference between UGSA &UNGSA on SC

Variables	UGSA		UNGSA		t	P
	M	SD	M	SD		
SC	27.4400	10.00685	25.4000	9.55334	2.085	.038

SC= Self-Confidence, UGSA= Urban Government School Adolescents,
UNGSA= Urban Non-Government School Adolescents

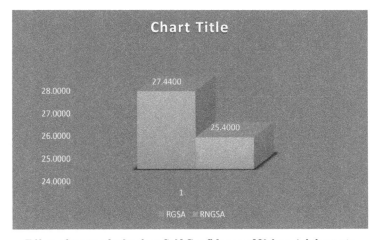

Effect of types of school on Self Confidence of Urban Adolescents

Table 4.119reveals that the calculated t value (2.085) is significant at 0.05 level of significance ($p<0.05$).It means that a significant difference is found between the self-confidence of UGSA and UNGSA on SC. It shows that types of School has a significant effect on SC of Urban Adolescents. The mean score of UGSA is 27.4400and UNGSA is 25.4000. The mean score of UGSA is greater than the mean score of UNGSA, in the present study more self-confidence score means less confidence and less self-confidence score means more confident. So the result indicate that UNGSA has more confident than UGSA. There is a great difference in the environment of government and non-government schools in urban areas. Non-government schools in urban area provide all facilities to the students as they charge heavy fees from them. They are able to provide a better academic environment. Whereas, government schools in urban areas fail to provide even the basic amenities to their students due to lack of funds. A good environment enhance the self-confidence. Therefore the self-confidence of UNGSA is higher than the UGSA.

i) **Comparison between government school and non-government school adolescents.**

TABLE- 4.120

Significance of difference between GSA & NGSA on SC

Variables	GSA		NGSA		T	P
	M	SD	M	SD		
SC	26.5600	10.30178	24.7925	9.43541	2.530	.012

GSA=Government school adolescents   NGSA=Non-government school adolescents

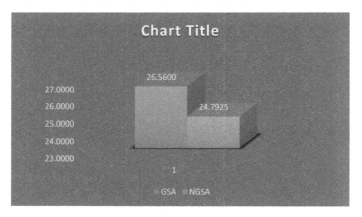

Effect of types of school on Self Confidence of Adolescents

A glance at Table 4.120 reveals that the calculated t value (2.530) which is significant at 0.05 level of significance ($p<0.05$). It means that a significant difference is found between the self-confidence of GSA and NGSA. It shows that types of School has a significant effect on SC of Adolescents. The mean score of GSA is 26.5600 and NGSA is 24.7925. The mean score of GSA is greater than the mean score of NGSA, in the present study more self-confidence score means less confidence and less self-confidence score means more confident. So the result indicate that NGSA has more confident than GSA.

It is quite evident that the school environment can help students developed qualities of character and citizenship and increase the behavior and self-confidence of the adolescents. Non- Government schools charge heavy fees from students, therefore they take the responsibility of all-round development of adolescents by providing them with proper facilities, opportunities and environment.

On the other hand government schools, due to lack of funds are unable to provide extra facilities to the students other than academics. That is why the confidence of NGSA is high. **Malhotra and Malhotra (2016)** revealed that gender, locality and type of school are associated with self-confidence.

PHASE IX (B)-The effect of types of school on Mental Health of adolescents.

a) **Comparison between government school and non-government school girl adolescents.**

TABLE- 4.121

Significance of difference between GSGA & NGSGA on MH

Variables	GSGA		NGSGA		t	P
	M	SD	M	SD		
MH	77.5400	9.35715	74.4700	8.73560	3.392	.001

MH= Mental Health, GSGA= Government School Girl Adolescents, NGSGA= Non-Government School Girl Adolescents

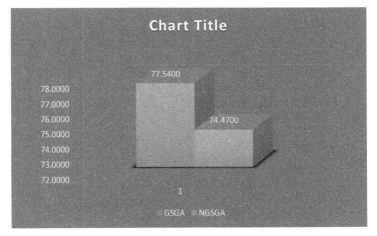

Effect of types of school on Mental Health of Girl Adolescents

Table 4.121reveals that the calculated t value (3.392) is significant at 0.01 level of significance (p<0.01).It means that a significant difference is found between the Mental Health of GSGA and NGSGA. It shows that types of School has a significant effect on MH of Girl Adolescents. The mean score of GSGA is 77.5400 and NGSGA is 74.4700. The mean score of GSGA is greater than the mean score of NGSGA, so the result indicate that GSGA has good mental health than NGSGA.

This may be due to the reason that, GSGA are better adjusted as compared to NGSGA. **Kukreti (1994)** reveled that girls studying in **Saraswati Vidhya Mandir (GS)** were better in all areas of adjustment. And **Srividhya, V., and Khadi, Pushpa, B.**

(2007) reveled that mental health was significantly correlated to adjustment problem, indicating the higher the problem lower the mental health. That is, those who have a low level of adjustment also have low mental health. Therefore the mental health of government schools girls is also good due to their good level of adjustment.

b) **Comparison between government school and non-government school boy adolescents.**

TABLE- 4.122

Significance of difference between GSBA & NGSBA on MH

Variables	GSBA		NGSBA		t	P
	M	SD	M	SD		
MH	76.0000	11.31282	74.0350	9.82734	1.854	.064

MH= Mental Health, GSBA= Government School Boy Adolescents, NGSBA= Non-Government School Boy Adolescents

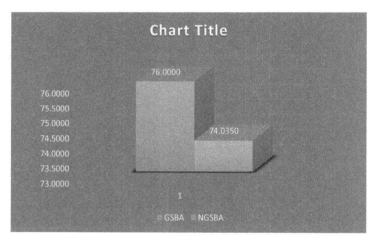

Effect of types of school on Mental Health of Boy Adolescents

A study of table 4.122 reveals that the calculated t value (1.854) is not significant at 0.05 level of significance (p>0.05). It means that there exist no significant difference between GSBA and NGSBA on MH. It shows that type of school does not effect on the MH of Boys Adolescents.

This may be because boys and girls are equally emotionally stable. The signs of an emotional stability may be cited as calmness of mind and freedom from anxiety and depression **(Hay and Ashman 2003)**. Emotional stability is a factor of mental health.

An emotionally stable person also has good mental health. **Kaur 2013**revealed that there was not any significant difference in various areas of emotional maturity of government and private school students. **Bindo 2016**also found that the students enrolled at the government and the private school have similar emotional stability level. Therefore there is no significant difference found between the mental health of GSBA and NGSBA.

c) **Comparison between rural government and non-government school girl adolescents.**

TABLE- 4.123

Significance of difference between RGSGA &RNGSGA on MH

Variables	RGSGA		RNGSGA		T	P
	M	SD	M	SD		
MH	76.0600	11.19598	73.1500	9.52972	1.979	.284

MH= Mental Health, RGSGA= Rural Government School Girl Adolescents,
RNGSGA= Rural Non-Government School Girl Adolescents

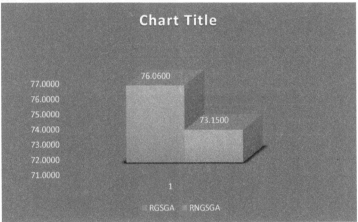

Effect of types of school on Mental Health of rural girl Adolescents

A careful inspection of Table 4.123reveals that the calculated t value (1.979) is not significant at 0.05 level of significance (p>0.05).It means that there exist no significant difference between RGSGA and RNGSGA on MH. It shows that type of school does not effect on the MH of Rural Girl Adolescents.

This might be due to the fact that there is not much difference in the environment of government and non-government schools in rural areas. The best adjusted adolescents belong to happy families where the adolescents and parents spend pleasurable time together and we know that rural areas are stress free as compared to urban areas. The adolescent girls learn to be adjustive emotionally, socially and educationally from their families and carry forward the same adjustment pattern to their school. And we know that adjustment level affect mental health also. **Srividhya, V., and Khadi, Pushpa, B. (2007)** reveled that mental health was significantly correlated to adjustment problem, indicating the higher the problem lower the mental health. That is, those who have a low level of adjustment also have low mental health. Therefore the mental health of government schools girls is also good due to their good level of adjustment. So, for girls from rural areas the type of school is not affecter that effect their mental health.

d) **Comparison between rural government and non-government school boy adolescents.**

TABLE- 4.124

Significance of difference between RGSBA &RNGSBA on MH

Variables	RGSBA		RNGSBA		t	P
	M	SD	M	SD		
MH	76.0600	11.19598	73.1500	9.52972	1.979	.049

MH= Mental Health, RGSBA= Rural Government School Boy Adolescents,
RNGSBA= Rural Non-Government School Boy Adolescents

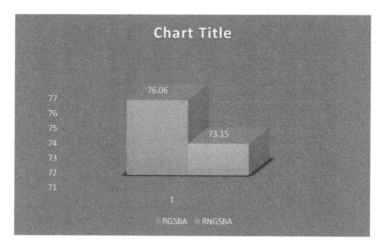

Effect of types of school on mental health of rural Boy Adolescents

A careful inspection of Table 4.124 reveals that the calculated t value (1.979) is significant at 0.05 level of significance ($p<0.05$). It means that a significant difference is found between the Mental Health of RGSBA and RNGSBA on MH. It shows that types of School has a significant effect on MH of Rural Boys Adolescents. The mean score of

RGSBA is 77.8600 and RNGSBA is 76.4800. The mean score of RGSBA is greater than the mean score of RNGSBA, so the result indicate that RGSBA has high mental health than from RNGSBA. The result is in congruence with the result of **Dr. Chitra Sharma 2017**revealing that the government school boys are more emotionally stable than the private school boys. Therefore the mental of RGSBA is higher than that of the RNGSBA.

e) **Comparison between urban government and non-government school girl adolescents.**

TABLE- 4.125

Significance of difference between UGSGA &UNGSGA on MH

Variables	UGSGA		UNGSGA		t	P
	M	SD	M	SD		
MH	77.2200	8.44899	72.4600	9.21069	3.808	.000

MH= Mental Health, UGSGA= Urban Government School Girl Adolescents,
UNGSGA= Urban Non-Government School Girl Adolescents

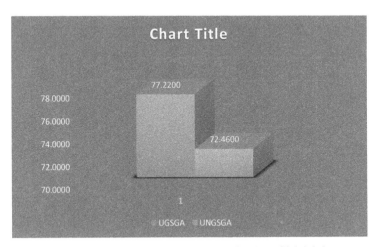

Effect of types of school on mental health of Urban Girl Adolescents

Observation of the Table 4.125shows that the calculated t value (3.808) which is significant at 0.01 level of significance (p<0.01).It means that a significant difference is found between the Mental Health of UGSGA and UNGSGA. It shows that types of School has a significant effect on MH of Urban Girl Adolescents. The mean score of

UGSGA is 77.2200 and UNGSGA is 72.4600. The mean score of UGSGA is greater than the mean score of UNGSGA, so the result indicate that UGSGA has good mental health than UNGSGA.

It may that UGSGA are better adjusted as compared to UNGSGA. Therefore the mental health of girl adolescents from non-government school of urban areas are higher than the girls from government school of urban areas.

f) **Comparison between urban government and non-government school boy adolescents.**

TABLE- 4.126

Significance of difference between UGSBA &UNGSBA on MH

Variables	UGSBA		UNGSBA		T	P
	M	SD	M	SD		
MH	75.9400	11.48457	74.9200	10.08617	.667	.505

MH= Mental Health, UGSBA= Urban Government School Boy Adolescents,
UNGSBA= Urban Non-Government School Boy Adolescents

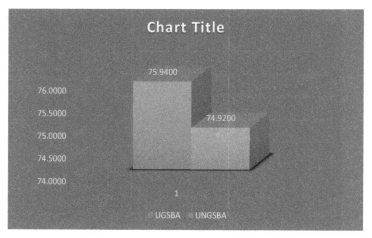

Effect of types of school on Mental Health of Urban Boy Adolescents

A study of Table 4.126revels that the calculated t value (.667) is not significant at 0.05 level of significance (p>0.05).It means that there exist no significant difference between UGSBA and UNGSBA on MH.

It shows that type of school does not affect the MH of Urban Boys Adolescents. The schools are poor or rich with respect to the environment they provide for their students. Among the various factors which contribute towards building the environment are classroom communication pattern, teaching strategies, motivation and rewards, spirit of competition, organizational setup etc. In urban areas both government school as well as non-government school try to provide the essential health environment to adolescents. Therefore there is no significant difference between the mental health of UGSBA and

UNGSBA.

g) **Comparison between Rural government and non-government school adolescents.**

TABLE- 4.127

Significance of difference between RGSA & RNGSA on MH

Variables	RGSA		RNGSA		t	P
	M	SD	M	SD		
MH	76.9600	10.72912	74.8150	8.83237	2.183	.030

MH=Mental Health, RGSA= Rural Government School Adolescents,
RNGSA= Rural Non-Government School Adolescents

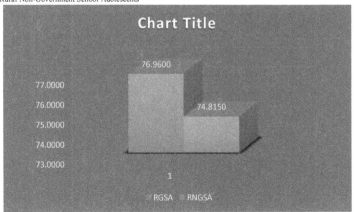

Effect of types of school on mental health of Rural Adolescents

A glance of Table 4.127 reveals the calculated t value (2.183) is significant at 0.05 level of significance ($p<0.05$). It means that a significant difference is found between the Mental Health of RGSA and RNGSA. It shows that types of School has a significant effect on MH of Rural Adolescents. The mean score of RGSA is 76.9600 and RNGSA is 74.8150. The mean score of RGSA is greater than the mean score of RNGSA, so the result indicate that RGSA has good mental health than RNGSA.

The result is in congruence with the result of **Dr. Chitra Sharma 2017** who shows that government school students are more emotionally stable then the private school students.

h) **Comparison between Urban government and non-government school adolescents.**

TABLE- 4.128

Significance of difference between UGSA &UNGSA on MH

Variables	UGSA		UNGSA		t	P
	M	SD	M	SD		
MH	76.5800	10.07677	73.6900	9.71265	2.920	.004

MH= Mental Health, UGSA= Urban Government School Adolescents,
UNGSA= Urban Non-Government School Adolescents

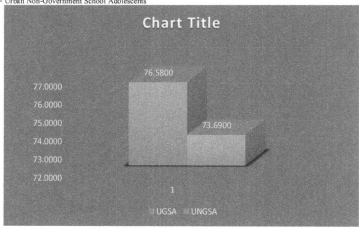

Effect of types of school on Mental Health of Urban Adolescents

A Perusal of Table 4.128 reveals that the calculated t value (2.920) is significant at 0.01 level of significance (p<0.01). It means that a significant difference is found between the Mental Health of UGSA and UNGSA. It shows that types of School has a significant effect on MH of Urban Adolescents. The mean score of UGSA is 76.5800 and UNGSA is 73.6900. The mean score of UGSA is greater than the mean score of UNGSA, so the result indicate that UGSA has good mental health than UNGSA.

The probable reason for the above result could be that the urban areas of Dehradun district is flooded with non-government schools where students from high SES come to study. The standard of most of these schools is very high where parents provide their wards with ample of money for the fulfillment of their needs. The urban pomp and show, distract the adolescent and they loss their self-control and adjustment level. On other hand UGSA have limited resources due to which they are not easily distracted towards the negativism of urban life style. Therefore the mental health of UGSA is higher than that of the UNGSA.

i) **Comparison between government school and non-government school adolescents.**

TABLE- 4.129

Significance of difference between GSA & NGSA on MH

Variables	GSA		NGSA		t	P
	M	SD	M	SD		
MH	76.7700	10.39675	74.2525	9.28840	3.612	.000

GSA=Government school adolescents   NGSA=Non-government school adolescents

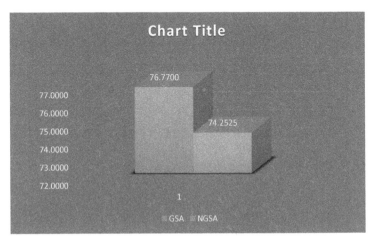

Effect of types of school on Mental Health of Adolescents

A glance of Table 4.129 reveals that the calculated t value (3.612) is significant at 0.01 level of significance (p<0.01).It means that a significant difference is found between the Mental Health of GSA and NGSA. It shows that types of School has a significant effect on MH of Adolescents. The mean score of GSA is 76.7700 and NGSA is 74.2525. The mean score of GSA is greater than the mean score of NGSA. So the result indicate that GSA has good mental health than NGSA.

The probable reason for the above result could be that most of the adolescents studying in non-government schools have high socio economic status. They pressurize their parents to provide them motor-cycle, heavy amount of pocket money to impress their friends etc.. They feel pride in smoking and are more prone to drug addiction. Due to which their mental health may be affected. On the other hand government school students have limited resources due to which they are not easily attracted towards the negativism of high SES life style. Due to which their mental health remains stable. Therefore the mental health of GSA is higher than the mental health of NGSA.

PHASE IX (C)-To find out the effect of types of school on the Personal Values of adolescents.

a) **Comparison between government school and non-government school girl adolescents.**

TABLE- 4.130

Significance of difference between GSGA & NGSGA on PV

Variables	GSGA		NGSGA		t	P
	M	SD	M	SD		
PV	137.3000	13.88358	129.9650	14.78230	5.115	.000

PV= Personal Values, GSGA= Government School Girl Adolescents, NGSGA= Non- Government School Girl Adolescents

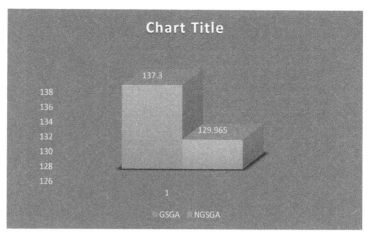

Effect of types of school on Personal Values of Girl Adolescents

A perusal of Table 4.130reveals that the calculated t value (5.115) is significant at 0.01 level of significance (p<0.01).It means that a significant difference is found between the Personal Values of GSGA and NGSGA. It shows that types of School has a significant effect on PV of Girls Adolescents. The mean score of GSGA is 137.3000 and NGSGA is 129.9650. The mean score of GSGA is greater than the mean score of NGSGA, so the result indicate that GSGA has more Personal values than NGSGA.

Adolescent girls spend most of their time either at home or in school. After family, the school environment also plays a significant role in the development of personal values in adolescents. In non-government school, much attention is not paid to the development of personal values of adolescents. **Dr. Mamta (2017)** found that the moral values of government school students is higher than the private school students.

b) **Comparison between government school and non-government school boy adolescents.**

TABLE- 4.131

Significance of difference between GSBA & NGSBA on PV

Variables	GSBA		NGSBA		t	P
	M	SD	M	SD		
PV	133.7950	18.34189	128.4500	16.20836	3.088	.002

PV= Personal Values, GSBA= Government School Boy Adolescents, NGSBA= Non- Government School Boy Adolescents

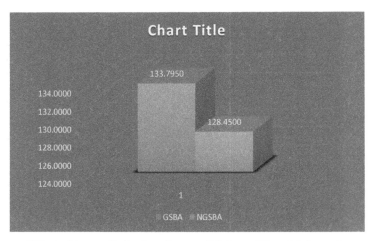

Effect of types of school on Personal Values of Boy Adolescents

A study of Table 4.131 reveals that the calculated t value (3.088) is significant at 0.01 level of significance (p<0.01). It means that a significant difference is found between the Personal Values of GSBA and NGSBA. It shows that types of School has a significant effect on PV of Boy Adolescents. The mean score of GSBA is 133.7950 and NGSBA is 128.4500. The mean score of GSBA is greater than the mean score of NGSBA, so the result indicate that GSBA has more personal values than NGSBA.

The probable reason for the above result could be that mostly non-government schools are available mostly in urban and semi-urban areas. The urban pomp and show distract the adolescents and they lose self-control and their personal values decline. On the other hand GSBA are not easily distracted toward the negativism of urban life style. The feeling of love, honesty, helpfulness etc. in them is greater than the boys of non-government schools.

c) **Comparison between rural government and non-government school girl adolescents.**

TABLE- 4.132

Significance of difference between RGSGA &RNGSGA on PV

Variables	RGSGA		RNGSGA		t	P
	M	SD	M	SD		
PV	138.0200	15.90564	134.4700	14.04427	1.673	.096

PV= Personal Values, RGSGA= Rural Government School Girl Adolescents,

RNGSGA= Rural Non-Government School Girl Adolescents

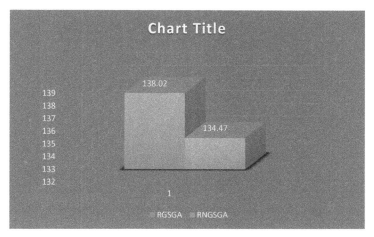

Effect of types of school on Personal Values of rural Girl Adolescents

The statistically calculated t value (1.673) is not significant at 0.05 level of significance (p>0.05). It means that there exist no significant difference between RGSGA and RNGSGA on PV. It shows that type of school has no effect on the PV of Rural Girl Adolescents.

d) **Comparison between rural government and non-government school boy adolescents.**

TABLE- 4.133

Significance of difference between RGSBA &RNGSBA on PV

Variables	RGSBA		RNGSBA		t	P
	M	SD	M	SD		
PV	133.9600	17.50089	126.0700	16.83626	3.249	.001

PV= Personal Values, RGSBA= Rural Government School Boy Adolescents,
RNGSBA= Rural Non-Government School Boy Adolescents

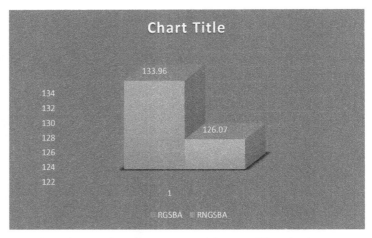

Effect of types of school on Personal Values of Boy Adolescents

The statistically calculated t value (3.249) is significant at 0.01 level of significance (p<0.01). It means that a significant difference is found between the Personal Values of RGSBA and RNGSBA. It means that types of School has a significant effect on PV of Rural Boy Adolescents. The mean score of RGSBA is 138.0200 and RNGSBA is 134.4700. The mean score of RGSBA is greater than the mean score of RNGSBA, so the result indicate that RGSBA have good personal values than RNGSBA.

e) **Comparison between urban government and non-government school girl adolescents.**

TABLE- 4.134

Significance of difference between UGSGA &UNGSGA on PV

Variables	UGSGA		UNGSGA		T	p
	M	SD	M	SD		
PV	136.5800	11.55066	125.4600	14.17739	6.081	.000

PV= Personal Values, UGSGA= Urban Government School Girl Adolescents,
UNGSGA= Urban Non-Government School Girl Adolescents

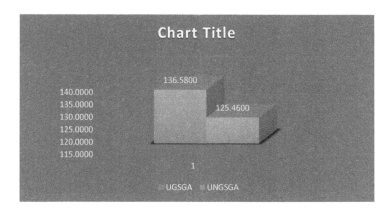

Effect of types of school on Personal Values of Urban Girl Adolescents

The statistically calculated t value (6.081) is significant at 0.01 level of significance (p<0.01). It means that a significant difference is found between the Personal Values of UGSGA and UNGSGA. It means that types of School has a significant effect on PV of Urban Girls Adolescents. The mean score of UGSGA is 136.5800 and UNGSGA is 125.4600. The mean score of UGSGA is greater than the mean score of UNGSGA, so the result indicate that UGSGA have good personal values than UNGSGA.

f) **Comparison between urban government and non-government school boy adolescents.**

TABLE- 4.135

Significance of difference between UGSBA &UNGSBA on PV

Variables	UGSBA		UNGSBA		t	P
	M	SD	M	SD		
PV	133.6300	19.23310	130.8300	15.27000	1.140	.256

PV= Personal Values, UGSBA= Urban Government School Boy Adolescents,
UNGSBA= Urban Non-Government School Boy Adolescents

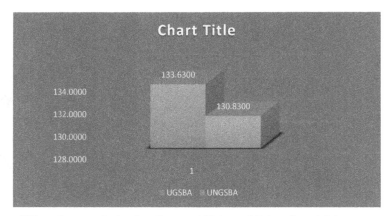

Effect of types of school on Personal Values of Urban Boy Adolescents

From the contents of Table 4.135 it is revealed that the calculated t value (1.140) is not significant at 0.05 level of significance (p>0.05).It means that there exist no significant difference between UGSBA and UNGSBA on PV. It shows that type of school does not affect the PV of Urban Boys Adolescents.

The reason for this may be that even though the school environment plays an important role in the development of personal values of adolescents. But in urban areas, the influence of urban life on the adolescents is so much that type of school has no effect on their personal values.

g) **Comparison between Rural government and non-government school adolescents.**

TABLE- 4.136

Significance of difference between RGSA &RNGSA on PV

Variables	RGSA		RNGSA		t	P
	M	SD	M	SD		
PVS	135.9900	16.80392	130.2700	16.02721	3.484	.001

PV= Personal Values, RGSA= Rural Government School Adolescents,
RNGSA= Rural Non-Government School Adolescents

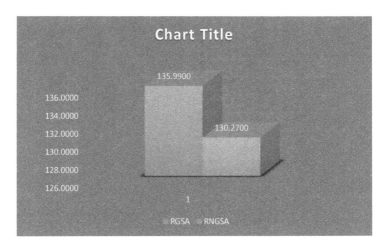

Effect of types of school on Personal Values of Rural Adolescents

A perusal of table 1.136 reveals that the calculated t value (3.484) is significant at 0.01 level of significance (p<0.01). It means that a significant difference is found between the Personal Values of RGSA and RNGSA on PV. It means that types of School has a significant effect on Rural Adolescents. The mean score of RGSA is 135.9900 and RNGSA is 130.2700. The mean score of RGSA is greater than the mean score of RNGSA, so the result indicate that RGSA has more Confident than RNGSA.

The result is in congruence with the study **Gupta (2002)** who found that there were significant difference in the values of students studying in government and private schools. **N. Rani (2009)** also confirmed that government school students have high moral values then private school students.

h) **Comparison between Urban government and non-government school adolescents.**

TABLE- 4.137

Significance of difference between UGSA &UNGSA on PV

Variables	UGSA		UNGSA		t	P
	M	SD	M	SD		
PV	135.1050	15.89298	128.1450	14.94122	4.512	.000

PV= Personal Values, UGSA= Urban Government School Adolescents,
UNGSA= Urban Non-Government School Adolescents

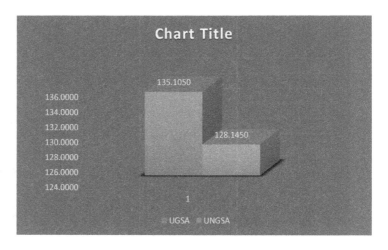

Effect of types of school on Personal Values of Urban Adolescents

From the content of Table 1.137 it is revealed that the calculated t value (4.512) is significant at 0.01 level of significance (p<0.01). It means that a significant difference is found between the Personal Values of UGSA and UNGSA. It means that types of School has a significant effect on PV of Urban Adolescents. The mean score of UGSA is 135.1050 and RNGSA is 128.1450. The mean score of UGSA is greater than the mean score of UNGSA, so the result indicate that UGSA have good personal values than UNGSA.

The result is in congruence with the finding **Malti (2006)** who found that the students of UP board schools have been found to have higher social and knowledge values than the students of CBSE board schools. **Dr. Mamta (2017)** revealed that there is a significant difference was found between the moral values of government and private school students. The moral values of government school students is higher than the private school students. The result also revealed that the female students have high moral values than male students of secondary school.

i) **Comparison between government and non-government school adolescents.**

TABLE- 4.138

Significance of difference between GSA &NGSA on PV

Variables	GSA		NGSA		t	P
	M	SD	M	SD		
PV	135.5475	16.34030	129.2075	15.51083	5.628	.000

GSA=Government school adolescents   NGSA=Non-government school adolescents

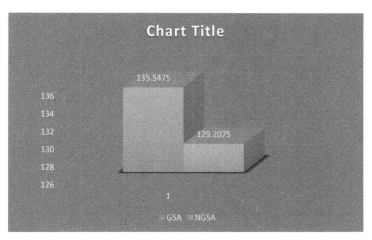

Effect of types of school on Personal Values of Adolescents

A glance at table 4.138 clearly reveals that the calculated t value (5.628) is significant at 0.01 level of significance (p<0.01). It means that a significant difference is found between the Personal Values of GSA and NGSA. It shows that types of School has a significant effect on PV of Adolescents. The mean score of GSA is 135.5475 and NGSA is 129.2075. The mean score of GSA is greater than the mean score of NGSA, so the result indicate that GSA has more Personal Values than NGSA.

The reason for this may be that most of the children studying in non-government schools belong to high SES families. Besides, more attention is paid to the academic achievement of the student in non-government schools. Whereas in government schools the environment is such that all the students live in harmony with each other and there is a feeling of love and cooperation in them. **N.Rani (2009)** revealed that government school students have high moral values then private school students.

Thus the results obtained from Tables 4.112 to 4.138 clarifies that type of school has a significant effect on self-confidence, mental health and personal values of adolescents. So the IX hypothesis predicting that, **"Type of school has null effect on Self-confidence, mental health and personal values of adolescents."** is rejected.

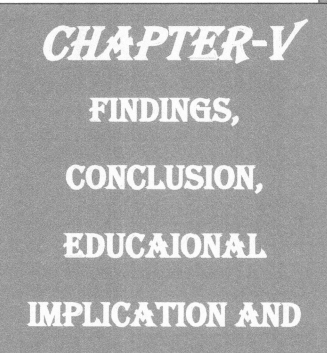

5.1 MAIN FINDINGS

1. **To find out the effect of different dimensions of socio-economic status of family on self-confidence of adolescents.**

   1.1 There exists a significant difference in the self-confidence of girl adolescents of different socio-economic levels. Those girl adolescents who belong to upper class are having high self-confidence than lower class SES girl adolescents.

   1.2 There exists a significant difference in the self-confidence of boy adolescents of different socio-economic levels. Those boy adolescents who belong to upper class are having high self-confidence than lower class SES boy adolescents.

   1.3 There exists a significant difference in the self-confidence of rural girl adolescents of different socio-economic levels. Those rural girl adolescents who belong to upper class are having high self-confidence than lower class SES rural girl adolescents.

   1.4 There exists a significant difference in the self-confidence of rural boy adolescents of different socio-economic levels. Those rural boy adolescents who belong to upper class are having high self-confidence than lower class SES rural boy adolescents.

   1.5 There exists no significant difference in the self-confidence of urban girl adolescents of different socio-economic levels.

   1.6 There exists a significant difference in the self-confidence of urban boy adolescents of different socio-economic levels. Those urban boy adolescents who belong to upper class are having high self-confidence than lower class SES urban boy adolescents.

   1.7 There exists no significant difference in the self-confidence of Government school girl adolescents of different socio-economic levels.

   1.8 There exists a significant difference in the self-confidence of government school boy adolescents of different socio-economic levels. Those government school boy adolescents who belong to upper class are having high self-confidence than lower class SES government school boy adolescents.

   1.9 There exists a significant difference in the self-confidence of non-government school girl adolescents of different socio-economic levels. Those non-government school girl adolescents who belong to upper class are having high self-confidence than lower class SES non-government school girl adolescents.

1.10 There exists a significant difference in the self-confidence of non-government school boy adolescents of different socio-economic levels. Those non-government school boy adolescents who belong to upper class are having high self-confidence than lower class SES non-government school boy adolescents.

1.11 There exists a significant difference in the self-confidence of adolescents of different socio-economic levels. Those adolescents who belong to upper class are having high self-confidence as compared to those who belong to lower class SES.

It has been observed that in case of boy adolescents significant difference was found in the self-confidence among different socio-economic levels of locality wise and type of school wise. On the other hand, for urban girl and government school girl adolescents no such significant difference has been observed.

Therefore, hypothesis I predicting that, **"There exists no significant difference between different dimension of socio-economic status and self-confidence of adolescents"** is partially rejected.

2. To find out the effect of different dimensions of socio-economic status of family on mental health of adolescents.

2.1 There exists a significant difference in the mental health of girl adolescents of different socio economic levels. Those girl adolescents who belong to upper class are having high mental health than those from the lower class.

2.2 There exists no significant difference in the mental health of boy adolescents of different socio economic levels.

2.3 There exists no significant difference in the mental health of rural girl adolescents of different socio economic levels.

2.4 There exists no significant difference in the mental health of rural boy adolescents of different socio economic levels.

2.5 There exists a significant difference in the mental health of urban girl adolescents of different socio economic levels. Those urban girl adolescents who belong to upper class are having high mental health than those from the lower class.

2.6 There exists no significant difference in the mental health of urban boy adolescents of different socio economic levels.

2.7 There exists no significant difference in the mental health of government school girl adolescents of different socio economic levels.

2.8 There exists no significant difference in the mental health of government school boy adolescents of different socio economic levels.

2.9 There exists no significant difference in the mental health of non- government school girl adolescents of different socio economic levels.

2.10 There exists no significant difference in the mental health of non-government school boy adolescents of different socio economic levels.

2.11 There exists a significant difference in the mental health of adolescents of different socio economic levels. Those adolescents who belong to upper class are having high mental health than those from the lower class.

Here we observed that in most of the cases the result was found to be non-significant difference. But in totality there exists a significant difference in the mental health of adolescents of different socio-economic status.

Thus the II Hypothesis predicting that **"There exists no significant difference of difference dimensions of socio-economic status on mental health of adolescents"** is partially rejected.

3. To find out the effect of different dimension of socio-economic status of family on personal values of adolescents.

3.1 There exists a significant difference in the personal values of girl adolescents of different socio economic levels. Those girl adolescents who belong to upper class are having good personal values than those from the lower class.

3.2 There exists a significant difference in the personal values of boy adolescents of different socio economic levels. Those boys' adolescents who belong to upper class are having good personal values than those from the lower class.

3.3 There exists a significant difference in the personal values of rural girl adolescents of different socio economic levels.

3.4 There exists a significant difference in the personal values of rural boy adolescents of different socio economic levels.

3.5 There exists a significant difference in the personal values of urban girl adolescents of different socio economic levels.

3.6 There exists no significant difference in the personal values of urban boy adolescents of different socio economic levels.

3.7 There exists no significant difference in the personal values of government school girl adolescents of different socio economic levels.

3.8 There exists a significant difference in the personal values of government school boy adolescents of different socio economic levels.

3.9 There exists a significant difference in the personal values of non-government school girl adolescents of different socio economic levels.

3.10 There exists no significant difference in the personal values of non-government school boy adolescents of different socio economic levels.

3.11 There exists a significant difference in the personal values of adolescents of different socio economic levels. Those adolescents who belong to upper class are having good persona values than those from the lower class.

Here we observed that in most of the cases the result was found to be significant difference. Thus the III Hypothesis predicting that **"There exists no significant difference of difference dimensions of socio-economic status on personal values of adolescents"** is partially rejected.

4. To see the relationship between self-confidence and mental health of adolescents.

4.1 Gender wise the relationship between self-confidence and mental health of adolescents is positively significant.

4.2 Locality wise relationship between self-confidence and mental health of girl adolescents is positively significant.

4.3 Locality wise relationship between self-confidence and mental health of boy adolescents is positively significant.

4.4 Positively significant relationship exists between self-confidence and mental health of rural girl adolescents on the basis of type of school.

4.5 Positively significant relationship exists between self-confidence and mental health of urban girl adolescents on the basis of type of school.

4.6 Positively significant relationship exists between self-confidence and mental health of rural boy adolescents on the basis of type of school.

4.7 Positively significant relationship exists between self-confidence and mental health of urban boy adolescents on the basis of type of school.

4.8 There exists a positive and highly significant relationship between self-confidence and mental health of adolescents.

Therefore hypothesis IV predicting that **"There exists no significant relationship between self-confident and mental health of adolescents"** is completely rejected.

5. To find the relationship between self-confidence and personal values of adolescents.

5.1 Both boy and girl adolescents have been found to have a positively significant relationship between their Self-Confidence and Personal Values.

5.2 A positively significant relationship is found between Self-Confidence and Personal Values of girl adolescents regardless of their locality.

5.3 A positively significant relationship is found between Self-Confidence and Personal Values of boy adolescents regardless of their locality.

5.4 A positively significant relationship is found between Self-Confidence and Personal Values of rural girl adolescents regardless of type of school.

5.5 A positively significant relationship is found between Self-Confidence and Personal Values of urban girl adolescents regardless of type of school.

5.6 A positively significant relationship is found between Self-Confidence and Personal Values of rural boy adolescents regardless of type of school.

5.7 A positively significant relationship is found between Self-Confidence and Personal Values of urban boy adolescents regardless of type of school.

5.8 It is found that a positive and highly significant relationship exists between Self-Confidence and Personal Values of adolescents.

Therefore hypothesis V predicting that **"There exists no significant difference between self-confidence and personal values of adolescents"** is completely rejected.

6. To find the relationship between mental health and personal values of adolescents.

6.1 Gender wise the relationship between MH and PV of adolescents is positively significant.

6.2 Locality wise relationship between MH and PV of girl adolescents is positively significant.

6.3 Locality wise relationship between MH and PV of boy adolescents is positively significant.

6.4 Positively significant relationship exists between mental health and personal values of rural girl adolescent on the basis of type of school.

6.5 Positively significant relationship exists between mental health and personal values of urban girl adolescent on the basis of type of school.

6.6 On the basis of type of school rural boy adolescent have a positively significant relationship between mental health and personal values.

6.7 On the basis of type of school urban boy adolescent have a positively significant relationship between mental health and personal values.

6.8 There exists a positive and highly significant relationship between mental health and personal values of adolescents.

Thus it has been found that regardless of locality, type of school or gender differences, there exists a positively significant relationship between mental health and personal values of adolescents. Therefore the null hypothesis VI predicting that **"there is no significant relationship between mental health and personal values of adolescents"** is completely rejected.

7 (A). To find out the effect of locality on the self-confidence of adolescents.

7.1 Significant difference exists between Rural and urban girl adolescent on self-confidence. The self-confidence of Rural Girls Adolescents is higher than Urban Girls Adolescents.

7.2. There is no significant difference found between rural and urban boy adolescents in relation to their self-confidence.

7.3 There is no significant difference found between rural and urban Government school girl adolescents in relation to their self-confidence.

7.4 There is no significant difference found between rural and urban Government school boy adolescents in relation to their self-confidence.

7.5 Significant difference exists between Rural and urban non-government school girl adolescent on self-confidence. The self-confidence of Rural Non-Government School Girl Adolescents is higher than Urban Non-Government School Girl Adolescents.

7.6. There is no significant difference found between rural and urban non- government school boy adolescents in relation to their self-confidence.

7.7 There is no significant difference found between rural and urban Government school adolescents in relation to their self-confidence.

7.8 There is no significant difference found between rural and urban Non-Government school adolescents in relation to their self-confidence.

7.9. No significant difference exists between Rural and Urban Adolescents on their self-confidence. It means that locality does not affect Self-confidence of adolescents.

7 (B). To find out the effect of locality on mental health of adolescents.

7.10 Significant difference exists between Rural and urban girl adolescent on mental health. The mental health of Rural Girl Adolescent is good than Urban Girl Adolescent.

7.11 There is no significant difference between rural and urban boy adolescent on mental health. It means that locality does not affect the mental health of boy adolescents.

7.12 There is no significant difference between rural and urban government school girl adolescent on mental health.

7.13 There is no significant difference between rural and urban government school boy adolescent on mental health.

7.14 Significant difference exists between rural and urban non-government school girl adolescents. The mental health of Rural Non-Government School Girl Adolescent is good than that of Urban Non-Government School Girl Adolescent.

7.15 There is no significant difference between rural and urban Non-government school boy adolescent on mental health.

7.16 There is no significant difference between rural and urban government school adolescent on mental health.

7.17 There is no significant difference between rural and urban non-government school adolescent on mental health.

7.18 There is no significant difference between rural and urban adolescent on mental health. It means that locality does not affect the mental health of adolescents.

7 (C). To find out the effect of locality on the personal values of adolescents.

7.19 There exists a significant difference between personal values of rural and urban girl adolescents. Rural girl adolescents have high personal values then urban girl adolescent.

7.20 No significant difference exists between Rural and Urban boy Adolescent on PV. It means that locality does not affect personal values of boy adolescents.

7.21 No significant difference exists between Rural and Urban Government School Girl Adolescents on PV. It means that locality does not affect personal values of Government school girl adolescents.

7.22 No significant difference exists between Rural and Urban Government School boy Adolescents on PV. It means that locality does not affect personal values of Government school boy adolescents.

7.23 There exists a significant difference between personal values of rural and urban non-government school girl adolescents. Rural non-government girl adolescents have high personal values then urban non- government school girl adolescent.

7.24 There exists a significant difference between personal values of rural and urban non-government school boy adolescents. Urban non-government boy adolescents have high personal values then Rural non- government school boy adolescent.

7.25 No significant difference exists between Rural and Urban Government School Adolescents on PV. It means that locality does not affect personal values of Government school adolescents.

7.26 No significant difference exists between Rural and Urban Non-Government School Adolescents on PV. It means that locality does not affect personal values of Non-Government school adolescents.

7.27 No significant difference exists between Rural and Urban Adolescents on their personal values. It means that locality does not affect personal values of adolescents.

Here we found that locality has no effect on self-confidence, mental health and personal values of adolescents. So the hypothesis VII predicting that **"Locality does not affect self-confidence, mental health and personal values of adolescents."** is accepted and we can say that Locality has non-significant effect on self-confidence, mental health and personal values of adolescents.

8 (A). To find out the effect of gender on the self-confidence of adolescents.

8.1 No significant difference exists between rural girl and boy adolescents on their self-confidence. It means that gender has no effect on self-confidence of rural adolescents.

8.2 Significant difference is obtained between urban girl and boy adolescents on their self-confidence. The result also found that urban boy adolescents have more confidence then urban girl adolescents.

8.3 No significant difference exists between rural government school girl and boy adolescents on their self-confidence.

8.4 No significant difference exists between urban government school girl and boy adolescents on their self-confidence.

8.5 Significant difference is obtained between rural non-government school girl and boy adolescents on their self-confidence. The result also found that rural non-government school girl adolescents have more confidence then rural non-government school boy adolescents.

8.6 Significant difference is obtained between urban non-government school girl and boy adolescents on their self-confidence. The result also found that urban non-government school boy adolescents have more confidence then urban non-government school girl adolescents.

8.7 No significant difference exists between government school girl and boy adolescents on their self-confidence.

8.8 No significant difference exists between non-government school girl and boy adolescents on their self-confidence.

8.9 No significant difference exists between girl and boy adolescents on their self-confidence. It means that gender has no effect on self-confidence of adolescents.

8 (B) To find out the effect of gender on the mental health of adolescents.

8.10 A significant difference exists between rural girl and boy adolescents on their mental health. The result also revealed that the rural girl adolescents have high mental health then that of rural boy adolescents.

8.11 There exists no significant difference between urban girl and boy adolescents on their mental health.

8.12 There exists no significant difference between rural government school girl and boy adolescents on their mental health.

8.13 There exists no significant difference between urban government school girl and boy adolescents on their mental health.

8.14 A significant difference exists between rural non- government school girl and boy adolescents on their mental health. The result also revealed that the rural non-government school girl adolescents have high mental health then that of rural non-government school boy adolescents.

8.15 There exists no significant difference between urban non-government school girl and boy adolescents on their mental health.

8.16 There exists no significant difference between government school girl and boy adolescents on their mental health.

8.17 There exists no significant difference between non-government school girl and boy adolescents on their mental health.

8.18 There exists no significant difference between girl and boy adolescents on their mental health.

8 (C). To find out the effect of gender on the personal values of adolescents.

8.19 A significant difference exists between rural girl and boy adolescents on their personal values. The result also revealed that the rural girl adolescents have more personal values then rural boy adolescents.

8.20 There exists no significant difference between urban girl and boy adolescents on their personal values.

8.21 There exists no significant difference between rural government school girl and boy adolescents on their personal values.

8.22 There exists no significant difference between urban government school girl and boy adolescents on their personal values.

8.23 A significant difference exists between rural non-government school girl and boy adolescents on their personal values. The result also revealed that the rural non-government school girl adolescents have more personal values then rural non-government school boy adolescents.

8.24 A significant difference exists between urban non-government school girl and boy adolescents on their personal values. The result also revealed that the urban non-government school boy adolescents have more personal values then urban non-government girl adolescents.

8.25 There exists significant difference between government school girl and boy adolescents on their personal values. The result also revealed that the government school girl adolescents have more personal values then government school boy adolescents.

8.26 There exists no significant difference between Non-government school girl and boy adolescents on their personal values.

8.27 A significant difference exists between girl and boy adolescents on their personal values. The result also revealed that the girl adolescents have more personal values then boy adolescents.

Here we found that gender has non-significant effect on self-confidence and mental health but a significant effect on personal values of adolescents. So the VIII hypothesis predicting **"No significant difference are obtained between self-confidence, mental health and personal values of adolescents when comparison is made on the basis of gender."** Is only partially accepted.

9 (A). To find out the effect of type of school on the self-confidence of adolescents.

9.1 There exists a significant difference between government and non-government school girl adolescents on their self-confidence. The non-government school girl adolescents are more self-confident then that of government school girl adolescents.

9.2 No significant difference exist between government and non-government school boy adolescents.

9.3 There exists a significant difference between government and non-government school rural girl adolescents on their self-confidence. The rural non-government school girl adolescents are more self-confident then that of rural government school girl adolescents.

9.4 No significant difference exist between rural government and non-government school boy adolescents.

9.5 No significant difference exist between urban government and non-government school girl adolescents.

9.6 There exists a significant difference between urban government and non-government school boy adolescents on their self-confidence. The urban non-government school boy adolescents are more self-confident then that of urban government school boy adolescents.

9.7 No significant difference exist between rural government and non-government school adolescents.

9.8 There exists a significant difference between urban government and non-government school adolescents on their self-confidence. The urban non-government school adolescents are more self-confident then that of urban government school adolescents.

9.9 There exists a significant difference between government and non-government school adolescents on their self-confidence. The non-government school adolescents are more self-confident then that of government school adolescents.

9 (B). <u>To find out the effect of type of school on the mental health of adolescents.</u>

9.10 There exists a significant difference between government and non-government school girl adolescents on their mental health. The result also revealed that government school girl adolescents have good mental health then non-government school girl adolescents.

9.11 No significant difference exist between government and non-government school boy adolescents.

9.12 No significant difference exist between rural government and non-government school girl adolescents.

9.13 There exists a significant difference between rural government and non-government school boy adolescents on their mental health. The result also revealed that rural government school boy adolescents have good mental health then rural non-government school boy adolescents.

9.14 There exists a significant difference between urban government and non-government school girl adolescents on their mental health. The result also revealed that urban government school girl adolescents have good mental health then urban non-government school girl adolescents.

9.15 No significant difference exist between urban government and non-government school boy adolescents.

9.16 There exists a significant difference between rural government and non-government school adolescents on their mental health. The result also revealed that rural government school adolescents have good mental health then rural non-government school adolescents.

9.17 There exists a significant difference between urban government and non-government school adolescents on their mental health. The result also revealed that urban government school adolescents have good mental health then urban non-government school adolescents.

9.18 There exists a significant difference between government and non-government school adolescents on their mental health. The result also revealed that government school adolescents have good mental health then non-government school adolescents.

9 (C). To find out the effect of type of school on the personal values of adolescents.

9.19 There exists a significant difference between government and non-government school girl adolescents on their personal values. The result also revealed that government school girl adolescents have good personal values then non-government school girl adolescents.

9.20 There exists a significant difference between government and non-government school boy adolescents on their personal values. The result also revealed that government school boy adolescents have good personal values then non-government school boy adolescents.

9.21 No significant difference exist between rural government and non-government school girl adolescents.

9.22 There exists a significant difference between rural government and non-government school boy adolescents on their personal values. The result also revealed that rural government school boy adolescents have good personal values then rural non-government school boy adolescents.

9.23 There exists a significant difference between urban government and non-government school girl adolescents on their personal values. The result also revealed that urban government school girl adolescents have good personal values then urban non-government school girl adolescents.

9.24 No significant difference exist between urban government and non-government school boy adolescents.

9.25 There exists a significant difference between rural government and non-government school adolescents on their personal values. The result also revealed that rural government school adolescents have good personal values then rural non-government school adolescents.

9.26 There exists a significant difference between urban government and non-government school adolescents on their personal values. The result also revealed that urban government school adolescents have good personal values then urban non-government school adolescents.

9.27 There exists a significant difference between government and non-government school adolescents on their personal values. The result also revealed that government school adolescents have good personal values then non-government school adolescents.

Here we found that type of school has a significant effect on self-confidence, mental health and personal values of adolescents. So the IX hypothesis predicting that, **"Type of school has null effect on Self-confidence, mental health and personal values of adolescents."** is rejected.

The main findings are on the basis of obtained data. It is also true that the family socio-economic status from low to high has deeply influenced various dimensions of adolescents' behaviour. Family is the fundamental unit of human society. All the members of the family together raise the level of the family. The development of a child starts from the family. From social, economic and educational outlook, role of the family is foremost. A family fulfils all the needs of the adolescents.

The main result of the present study reveals that the adolescents from different socio-economic status have differences in their self-confidence, mental health and personal values. The results further showed that adolescents from high socio-economic status had higher self-confidence, mental health and personal values in comparison to adolescents from low socio-economic status. The reason for this may be that despite Dehradun being a big city of uttarakhand, families of different socio-economic status are found here. There are many big government and private offices in which there are big officers whose socio economic status is high, but the socio-economic status of the people working in lower classes of these offices is low. Although the sample selection was done from both ruler as well as urban areas, from government as well as non-government schools from girls as well as boys adolescents still, in totality their family socio-economic status turned out to be either high, moderate or low.

Adolescents are the future citizens of the country. It is the duty of parents and families to turn adolescents in to healthy and noble citizens. They are not only the future of the nation but also its strength in reserve. Family is responsible for the development of self-confidence, mental health and personal values in adolescents.

Present study has more behavioural importance. On the basis of the result of the study families will easily understand their duties and responsibilities towards their adolescents. Self-confidence, mental health and personal values are important factor of personality and they have an important role in the development of the adolescents. Self-confidence encourage a person to do any work. The mental health of a person helps him to adjust to his environment and his personal values help him to distinguish between good and bad. Therefore, concrete steps should be taken to develop the self-confidence, mental health and personal values of the adolescents.

Positive relationship between families and adolescents is important because it builds the feeling of self-respect and confidence. It gives an individual the courage to meet the challenges of life and permits him to utilize his experiences constructively. Families should provide healthy environment to adolescents so that they become confident, mentally health and personally valued.

5.2 CONCLUSION

The conclusion is important for the investigation as it gives the final shape to the work. It allows to summaries ideas, to summaries the importance of ideas and to inspire readers for new perspectives. Conclusion is a subject of investigation and have an important place. The conclusions based on the analysis and interpretation of the data are presented below.

The study found differences in self-confidence, mental health and personal values among adolescents with different socio-economic status. The results further showed that adolescents with high socio-economic status had higher self-confidence, mental health and personal values than adolescents with lower socio-economic status. A positive and significant relation was found between adolescent's self-confidence and mental health; Self-Confidence and personal values; Personal Values and Mental health.

It was further revealed that no difference was found in the self-confidence, mental health and personal values of rural as well as urban adolescents. But the self-confidence and personal values of the girls in rural areas was higher than the girls in urban areas whereas the mental health of urban girl adolescents was higher than that of rural girl adolescents. The mental health and personal values and self-confidence of girls studying in non-government school of rural areas was higher than girls studying in non-government schools of urban areas.

The study also revealed that while there was no difference in Self-confidence and mental health of girl and boy, but girl had high personal values than boys. The self-confidence of urban boys and the mental health of rural girls were respectively higher than that of urban girls and the mental health of rural boys. It was further found that self-confidence and mental health of girls studying in non-government schools in rural areas was higher than that of boys.

The study further revealed that the self-confidence of adolescence studying in non-government schools was higher than that of adolescence studying in government schools. But their mental health and personal values were lower than that of adolescents from govt. schools.

In short, it can be said that gender, and locality had no effect on adolescent's self-confidence and mental health, but the adolescent's personal values were influenced by Gender. The type of school had an impact on adolescent's self-confidence, mental health and personal values.

5.3 EDUCATIONAL IMPLICATIONS

1. The findings of the present study have important implications for teachers, parents, institutions and for educational and schools counselors to perform their respective job well.

2. The findings of this study will help to overcome the problems of gender difference, locality, school environment and socio-economic status which influence the self-confidence, mental health and personal values of adolescents.
3. Findings make a significant contribution to improving self-confidence mental health and personal values among adolescents.
4. The findings will also help teachers and parents to understand the importance of high self-confidence and good personal values in reducing mental disorders like anxiety, stress, emotional instability, depression in adolescence.
5. The finding will help family members to understand the importance of the home environment in enhancing adolescent's self-confidence, mental health and personal values, as their have being found a positive relationship with socio-economic status of family.
6. As a positive relationship has been found between self-confidence, mental health and personal values, this study will enable psychologists and counsellors to reduce mental problems arising among adolescent.
7. The results obtained can be used to understand that adolescents success can be influenced not only by his intelligence but also by his self-confidence, mental health and personal values.
8. The findings of the study can also be helpful for giving proper guidance and counselling to parents and their adolescents.
9. The results obtained may inspire policy makers to formulate such policies that reduce variations in the school environment as the study found that the type of school had an impact on adolescent's self-confidence, mental health and personal values.
10. The findings of the present study will also help to school administration to organize mental health programs which will focus on promoting mental wellness, preventing mental health problems and providing treatment.
11. The findings of the present study will help to recognize those circumstances in which adolescents experience mental health problems.

5.4 SUGGESTION

5.4.1. SUGGESTION FOR FUTURE STUDY

1. In the present study only the students of Dehradun district have been taken for further study a comparison can be made between the students of any two districts.

2. Difference in the home environment may be analyzed for different socio-economic status families.

3. Difference in the different dimensions of mental health may be analyzed for different socio-economic status families.

4. A variety of values like spiritual values, domestic values, moral values, social values etc. can be analyzed among adolescents from families with different socio-economic status.

5. The impact of joint family and nuclear family can be seen on the child's self-confidence, mental health and personal values.

7. Other factors affecting self-confidence, mental health and personal values can also be studied.

8. The study can be done at different levels of education i.e. at primary level, elementary level, secondary school level and higher education level.

9. The effect of working and non-working mother on the self-confidence, mental health and personal values could be undertaken.

10. Adolescents from different blocks of Dehradun district can be compared in their self-confidence, mental health and personal values.

11. The impact of different component of SES can be seen individually such as the impact of education of parents on SC, MH and PV of adolescents.

5.4.2 SUGGESTION FOR PARENTS

1. Adolescence is a difficulty period of development. So at this stage, it is the responsibility of the parents to understand the problems of the adolescents.

2. Parents should behave friendly with the adolescents so that they can share their problems with them.

3. Parents should encouraged adolescents. They should be thought to recognized right and wrong and inculcate good values in them.

4. Parent should put pressure on adolescents to study according to their ability, otherwise it can created stress, anxiety, depression etc. In them.

5. Parents should pay attention to the activities of the adolescents so as to prevent the development of bad habits in them.

6. Parents should change their old perceptions and think according to the thoughts of new generation to reduce generation gap in them.

7. Parents should acknowledge adolescents' feelings and show them that you understand them.

8. Parents can inculcate good values by becoming role models for the adolescents.

9. Parents should spend quality time with them and create an environment where they feel comfortable to explore.

10. Parents should encourage to their child to helping others.

11. As a parents you should want to make sure that your child's learning environment is to set in such a way so that they can successful in their life.

12. Parents should make sure that their child gain love and care.

5.4.3 SUGGESTION FOR TEACHER

1. Teacher should help in reducing the feeling of failure in adolescents so that the self-confidence of them can be enhanced.

2. The teacher should encouraged the adolescents to perform better in life.

3. Teachers can inculcate good values by becoming role models for the students.

4. The teachers should guide the students for the future.

5. Teacher should use such extra-curricular activities, which enhance the confidence level of students and make them mentally healthy.

6. Teachers should be found out the mental health problems of students.

7. Teachers should promote the social and emotional competency of students.

8. Teachers should reinforce positive behavior and decision making power in students.

9. Teachers should learn more about ways to support their students.

10. Teachers should help to their students to recognize mental health issues.

11. Teachers should send this healthy message to their students that their self-worth is not based on their grades, their mental well-being is just as important as a academic performance.

5.4.4 SUGGESTION FOR ADOLESCENTS

1. Adolescents should follow the guidelines given by their parents and teachers.

2. Adolescents should learn to adjust in all situation, which helps them to stay mentally healthy.

3. They should maintain their self-confidence in any circumstances of life.

4. They should avoid the consumption of things like smoking, intoxication, drugs etc. as it can cause many mental disorders in them.

5. They should adopt good habits like honesty, punctuality, helpfulness, cleanliness, discipline etc.

6. Adolescents should be learn to maintain their trust among the family members.

5.4.5 SUGGESTION FOR POLICY MAKER, ADMINISTRATORS AND EDUCATIONISTS

1. Policymakers can minimize the problem of adolescents related to gender difference and socio-economic status by conducting seminars and workshop, which enhance the self-confidence, mental health and personal values of adolescents.

2. Such co-curricular activities should be included in the curriculum, which reduce the academic pressure and rise up the confidence in the students.

3. From time to time, programs related to guidance and counselling for adolescents should be organized by school administration.

4. Value education should be included in the curriculum up to the higher secondary level.

5. It is very necessary that we teach our adolescents to live in harmony and peace and make them good citizen.

6. From time to time the school administration should educate their staff, students and their parents on symptoms of and help for mental health problems.

7. There should be counselors and psychologist in every school.

CPSIA information can be obtained
at www.ICGtesting.com
Printed in the USA
LVHW060755040623
748794LV00030B/165